ALLE ZEIT WACH 1842

Detection of Ischemic Myocardium with Exercise

Edited by

F. Loogen and L. Seipel

With 115 Figures

Springer-Verlag
Berlin Heidelberg New York 1982

Professor Dr. med. Franz Loogen
Medizinische Klinik B
Universität
Moorenstr. 5
D-4000 Düsseldorf, FRG

Professor Dr. med. Ludger Seipel
Medizinische Klinik III
Medizinische Universitätsklinik
D-7400 Tübingen, FRG

Proceedings of an International Symposium held in Düsseldorf, February 28 - March 1, 1980

ISBN-13:978-3-642-68389-3 e-ISBN-13:978-3-642-68387-9
DOI: 10.1007/978-3-642-68387-9

Library of Congress Cataloging in Publication Data
Main entry under title: Detection of ischemic myocardium with exercise. „Proceedings of an international symposium held in Düsseldorf, February 28-March 1, 1980"--Verso t.p. Includes bibliographies. 1. Coronary heart disease--Diagnosis--Congresses. 2. Exercise tests--Congresses. I. Loogen, F. (Franz), 1919- . II. Seipel, L. [DNLM: 1. Coronary disease --Diagnosis. 2. Exercise test. WG 300 D479] RC685.C6D456 616.1'237075
81-23221
ISBN-13:978-3-642-68389-3 (U.S.) AACR2

Softcover reprint of the hardcover 1st edition 1982

2119/3140-543210

Preface

The detection of ischemic myocardium is one of the major problems in modern cardiology. Exercise has long been used to detect latent myocardial ischemia by enhancing oxygen demand, but different cardiologists perform exercise tests in different ways. In addition, many new techniques for detection of ischemia have been developed in the past decade. For these reasons, a symposium on this topic was organized in Düsseldorf under the auspices of the European Society of Cardiology.

The papers from this symposium contained herein provide an up-to-date review of the different forms of exercise tests, including their advantages and disadvantages. Indications for study, recording techniques and evaluation of exercise ECG, including computer techniques, are extensively discussed. The results of exercise ECG are compared with those of other methods, especially coronary angiography. Finally, the prognostic value of exercise ECG is assessed. Additional chapters deal with complementary methods for detection of myocardial ischemia, presenting techniques and results of angiographic, isotopic and metabolic studies under exercise.

The symposium demonstrates that exercise testing has a primary role in the detection of the disease, but there is still no unanimity on how to carry it out. The results of some new approaches are promising, even if their clinical relevance has not yet been fully established. We hope that this book will be of interest to all our colleagues taking care of cardiac patients.

We wish especially to thank Mr. M. Gücker and Mrs. B. Kratzenberg of Pharma-Schwarz Inc., Monheim, for their tremendous organizational and practical contribution to the planning of the meeting in Düsseldorf. Only the financial support of Pharma-Schwarz made the symposium and the publication of the proceedings possible.

F. Loogen
L. Seipel

Contents

Part I
Exercise Testing 1

Forms of Exercise Testing
M. Kaltenbach 3

Exercise Protocol
A. Holmgren and T. Ivert 9

The Optimal Lead System for Detection of Ischemic Myocardium
M. Niederberger and S. Panzer 19

Variations in Data of Exercise Tests due to External and Environmental Conditions
J.P. Broustet, P. Guern, J.F. Cherrier, M. Sicart, and P.M. Neuville 23

Evaluation of ECG Changes
B. Caru, S. Pirelli, C. Candotti, G. Cattafi, A. Manzini, and M. Mangiavacchi 34

The Clinical Value of Computer Assistance in the Exercise Laboratory
M.L. Simoons, R. Vinke, S. Mey, and P.G. Hugenholtz 38

The Value of Holter Monitoring for Detection of Ischemic Heart Disease
M.L. Simoons, T. Boehmer, J. Roelandt, and J. Pool 43

Telemetry
K. Bachmann, G. Raab, and R. Zerzawy 49

Value of Additional Measurements During Exercise Testing: Oxygen Consumption, Blood Pressure, and Cardiac Output
J.M.R. Detry, P. Mairiaux, K. Kandouci, P. Mengeot, J. Melin, and M.F. Rosseau 58

Indications for Electrocardiographic Exercise Testing in the Detection of Ischemic Myocardium
M.H. Frick 72

Prognostic Value of Stress Testing
M.H. Ellestad 77

Part II
Coronary Angiography and Ventriculography 85

Methodology of Coronary Angiography and Ventriculography
with Special Reference to Exercise
U. Gleichmann, G. Trieb, U. Sigwart, H. Mannebach, and
D. Fassbender 87

Relationship Between Coronary Obstructions and Regional Myocardial
Blood Flow in Man During Stress Provoked by Rapid Atrial Pacing
P.R. Lichtlen and H.J. Engel 98

Part III
ECG and Coronarography 111

Comparison of Exercise ECG and Coronary Angiography
H. Rosskamm and L. Samek 113

Studies in Patients with Abnormal Electrocardiogram of
Unknown Etiology
H. Kuhn, B. Lösse, and W. Hort 122

Ventricular Arrhythmias and Angiographic Findings
K.P. Bethge and P.R. Lichtlen 125

Part IV
Complementary Methods 135

Analysis of Drug Effects on Left Ventricular Isovolumic Contraction
During Atrial Pacing
P.W. Serruys, R.W. Brower, J. Lubsen, M.v.d. Brand, G.T. Meester,
and P.G. Hugenholtz 137

Interest of Gamma-Angiocardiography at Rest, After Leg Raising, and
After Nitroglycerin in Coronary Artery Disease and Myocardial Infarction
M. Brochier, T. Planiol, R. Itti, B. Charbonnier, P. Raynaud,
and J. Helias 151

Thallium Scintigraphy
H. Schicha, P. Retrop, K.R. Karsch, L. Facorro, H. Blanke, H. Kreutzer,
and D. Emrich 156

Myocardial Scintigraphy with Free Fatty Acids and Glucose
K. Vyska, C. Freundlieb, A. Höck, L.E. Feinendegen, G. Kloster,
H.J. Machulla, and G. Stöcklin 165

Exercise and Myocardial Ischemia in Patients with Angina Pectoris
A.P. Selwyn, K.M. Fox, R. Allan, A. Jonathan, and T. Jones 173

Detection of Ischemic Myocardium with Exercise: Coronary Blood
Flow Measurements
W. Kübler, D. Opherk, and H. Zebe 184

List of Authors and Chairmen

Professor Dr. K. Bachmann
Medizinische Poliklinik der Universität
Östliche Stadtmauerstraße 29
D-8520 Erlangen, FRG

R.Balcon, M.D.
Fullham Road
London SW 36 HP, U.K.

Dr. K.-P. Bethge
Medizinische Hochschule
Abteilung für Kardiologie
Karl-Wiechert-Allee 9
D-3000 Hannover 61, FRG

Professor Dr. H. Blömer
I. Medizinische Klinik
Technische Universität
Klinikum rechts der Isar
Ismaninger Straße 22
D-8000 München 80, FRG

Professor Dr. M. Brochier
Centre Hospitalier Regional de Tours
Clinique Cardiologique
2, Boulevard Tonnelle
F-37033 Tours Cedex, France

Professor Dr. J.-P. Broustet
Hopital Cardiologique du Haut Leveque
Avenue de Magellan
F-33604 Bordeaux, France

Dr. B. Caru
Via Ippodromo 9
I-20151 Milano, Italy

Professor Dr. M. Degeorges
Hopital Cochin
27, rue du Faubourg St. Jacques
F-75014 Paris, France

Professor Dr. H. Denolin
178, Av. Winston Churchill
Boite 10
B-1180 Bruxelles, Belgium

Dr. J.M. Detry
Laboratoire d'Exploration Fonctionelle
Cardio-pulmonaire
Cliniques Universitaires St. Pierre
Brusselsestraat 69
B-3000 Leuven, Belgium

M.H. Ellestad, M.D.
Memorial Hospital Medical Center
2801 Atlantic Avenue
P.O. Box 1428
Long Beach, California 90801, USA

Professor Dr. L.E. Feinendegen
Medizinische Klinik
Kernforschungsanlage Jülich GmbH
Postfach 1913
D-5170 Jülich, FRG

Professor Dr. M.H. Frick
Helsinki University
Central Hospital
Cardiovascular Laboratory
First Department of Medicine
Hartmaninkatur 4
SF-00290 Helsinki 29, Finland

Professor Dr. U. Gleichmann
Gollwitzer-Meier-Institut
Klinik für Herz- und Kreislauferkrankungen
Herforder Straße 43
D-4970 Bad Oeynhausen, FRG

Professor Dr. A. Holmgren
Clinical Phys. Laboratory
Thoracic Clinics
Karolinska Hospital
S-10401 Stockholm, Sweden

Professor Dr. W. Hort
Pathologisches Institut der Universität
Moorenstraße 5
D-4000 Düsseldorf, FRG

Professor Dr. P.G. Hugenholtz
Thoraxcenter
Medizinische Faculteit
Postbus 1738
NL-3000 Rotterdam, The Netherlands

Professor Dr. M. Kaltenbach
Abteilung für Kardiologie
Zentrum Innere Medizin der Universität
Theodor-Stern-Kai 7
D-6000 Frankfurt a.M. 70, FRG

Professor Dr. W. Kübler
Medizinische Universitätsklinik
Kardiologie
Bergheimer Straße 58
D-6900 Heidelberg 1, FRG

Professor Dr. H.Kuhn
Medizinische Klinik B der Universität
Kardiologie
Moorenstraße 5
D-4000 Düsseldorf, FRG

Professor Dr. P.R. Lichtlen
Medizinische Hochschule
Abteilung für Kardiologie
Karl-Wiechert-Allee 9
D-3000 Hannover 61, FRG

P D Dr. B.Lösse
Medizinische Klinik B der Universität
Kardiologie
Moorenstraße 5
D-4000 Düsseldorf, FRG

Professor Dr. F. Loogen
Medizinische Klinik B der Universität
Kardiologie
Moorenstraße 5
D-4000 Düsseldorf, FRG

Professor Dr. A.Maseri
Hammersmith Hospital
Ducane Road
London W 12 OHS, U.K

Universitätsdozent Dr. E. Niederberger
Kardiologische Universitätsklinik
Garnisonsgasse 13
A-1090 Wien, Austria

Dr. J. Roelandt
Erasmus Universiteit
Postbus 1738
NL-3000 DR Rotterdam, The Netherlands

Professor Dr. H. Roskamm
Benedikt Krankenhaus
Südring 15
D-7812 Bad Krozingen, FRG

Privatdozent Dr. H. Schicha
Institut für Nuklearmedizin der Universität
D-3400 Göttingen, FRG

Professor Dr. L. Seipel
Medizinische Klinik III, Universitätsklinik
D-7400 Tübingen, FRG

A.Selwyn, M.D.
University of London
Royal Postgraduate Medical School
Hammersmith Hospital
Ducane Road
London W 12 OHS, U.K.

Dr. P.Serruys
Academisch Ziekenhuis
Ziekenhuis Dijkzigt
Dr. Molewaterplein 40
NL-3015 Rotterdam, The Netherlands

Dr. M.L. Simoons
Erasmus Universiteit
Postbus 1738
NL-3000 DR Rotterdam, The Netherlands

Dr. E. Varnauskas
Medical University Hospital
Department of Cardiology
S-Gothenburg, Sweden

PD Dr. K.Vyska
Institut für Medizin
Kernforschungsanlage Jülich GmbH
Postfach 1913
D-5170 Jülich 1, FRG

Part I
Exercise Testing

Forms of Exercise Testing

M. Kaltenbach

Many forms of exercise have been used to determine human physical capacity. Within the last few decades most of the seven forms shown in Fig. 1 have been in use. No standardization has been achieved yet, however. In the following text four different types will be compared in order to show the similarities and the essential differences.

Even if identical physical work is performed, the biologic response is different. Turning a bicycle with the legs requires less energy than doing the same work with both arms [3]. Riding a bicycle in a sitting position leads to 20% less increase in left ventricular filling pressure as compared to the same bicycle work performed in the supine position. Therefore, to achieve comparable biologic results, not only the physical work load, but also the type of exercise and the body position in which the work has been performed have to be defined.

Ideally, a linear relationship exists between physical work load and energy consumption over a wide range of physical load. In Fig. 2 this relationship is shown for bicycle as well as for special form of step test.

The reproducibility of exercise test is rather good if the same person performs the same work on the same ergometer (Fig. 3). If, however, different instruments are used,

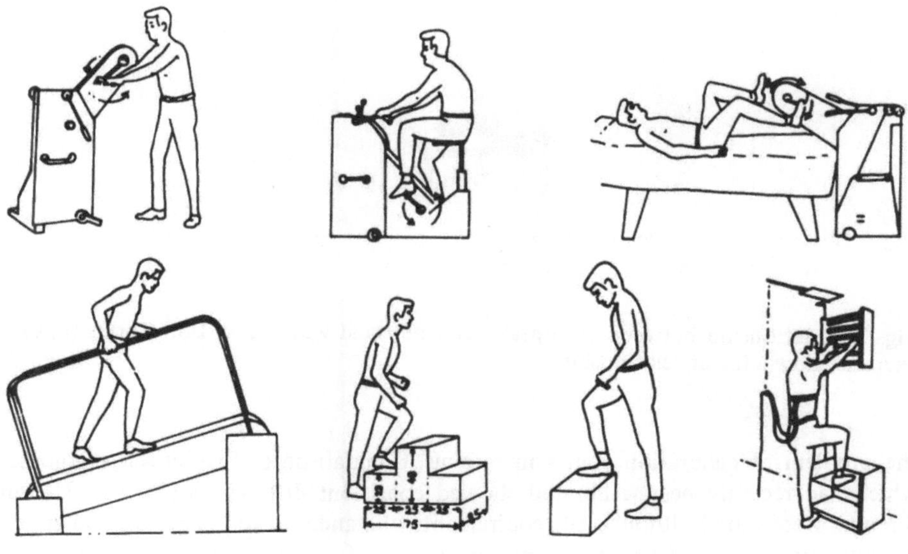

Fig. 1. Seven different forms of exercise testing

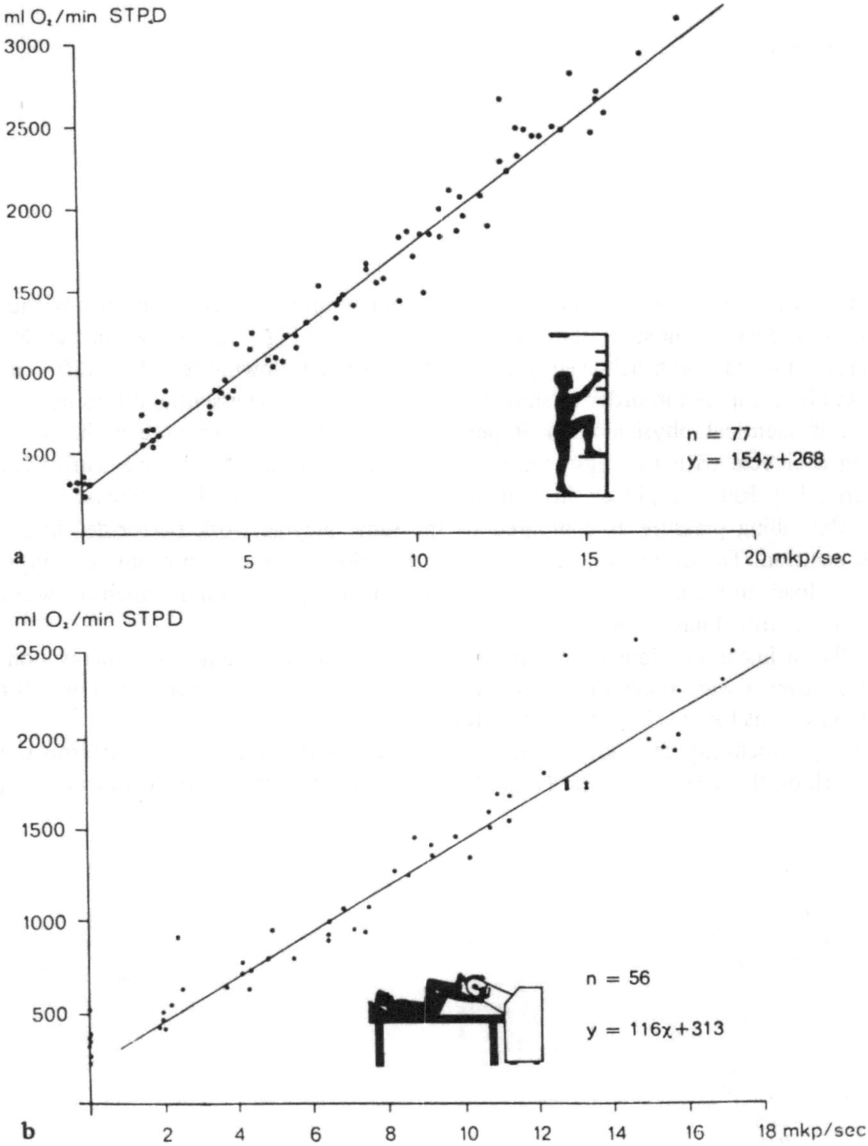

Fig. 2. Relationship between O_2 uptake and physical work load. Both forms (**a, b**) of exercise show a linear relationship

the problem of calibration comes into focus. Comparison of five bicycle ergometers which had recently been calibrated showed consistent differences (Fig. 4). The differences were found although all requirements of standardization had been taken into consideration, such as speed of rotation, length of pedals, and rotating mass. This calibration problem is not present in types of work such as the step test or treadmill.

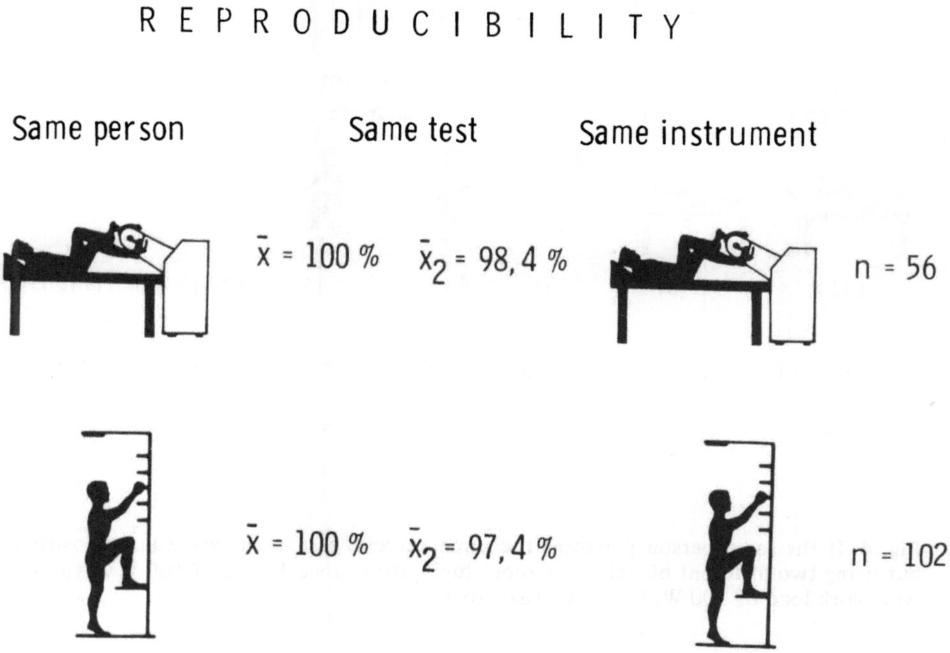

Fig. 3. If the same person performs the same exercise test in the same body position using the same instrument, the reproducibility is satisfactory

Specific aims of exercise tests can only be achieved with certain forms of exercise. During left or right heart catheterization, for example, bicycle work can best be performed in the supine position. In the sitting position the zero leveling of the pressure transducer is more difficult. For the early detection of myocardial ischemia on the other hand, bicycle ergometry is limited by the fact that leg pain and general fatigue often occur before the coronary reserve in a given patient is exhausted. Particularly in patients with less severe forms of angina pectoris bicycle work often has to be stopped due to muscle fatigue at a point at which coronary circulation would have allowed the continuation of exercise. Comparison of bicycle work with a specific form of step test shows a highly significant increase in tolerated working time if the patient performs the work with larger muscle mass (Fig. 5).

In clinical practice exercise tests are mostly done to demonstrate or to exclude ischemic changes in the electrocardiogram during and after exercise. Demonstration of myocardial ischemia in patients with severe angina requires low exercise loads and can be achieved with any kind of exercise. Demonstration of less severe ischemia or exclusion of coronary heart disease, however, requires high work loads and is best done with tests involving large muscle mass.

The form of exercise as well as the body position can influence the complication rate and therefore has to be taken into consideration when different forms are recommended. A survey done in German-speaking European countries covered a total of more than 1 million exercise tests, among them over 700 000 involving patients with

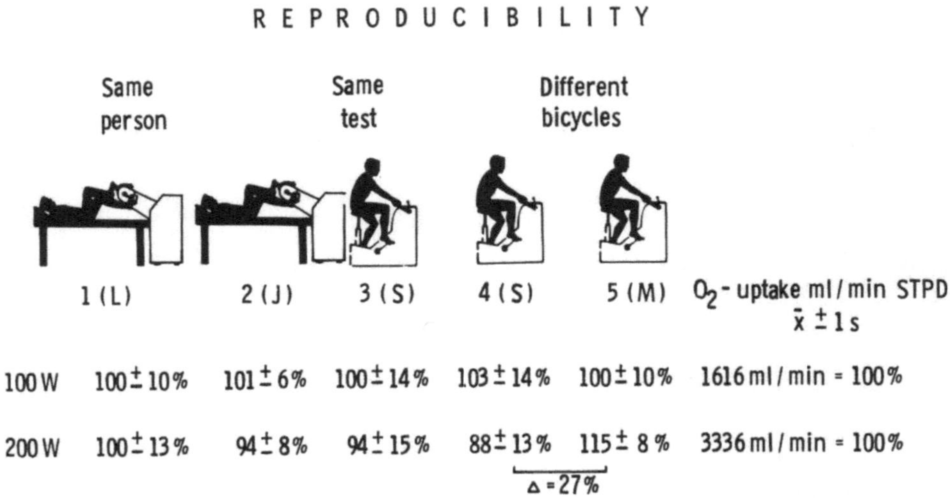

Fig. 4. If the same person performs the same exercise test in the same body position but using two different bicycles, the reproducibility at a work load of 100 W was good. At a work load of 200 W it was unsatisfactory

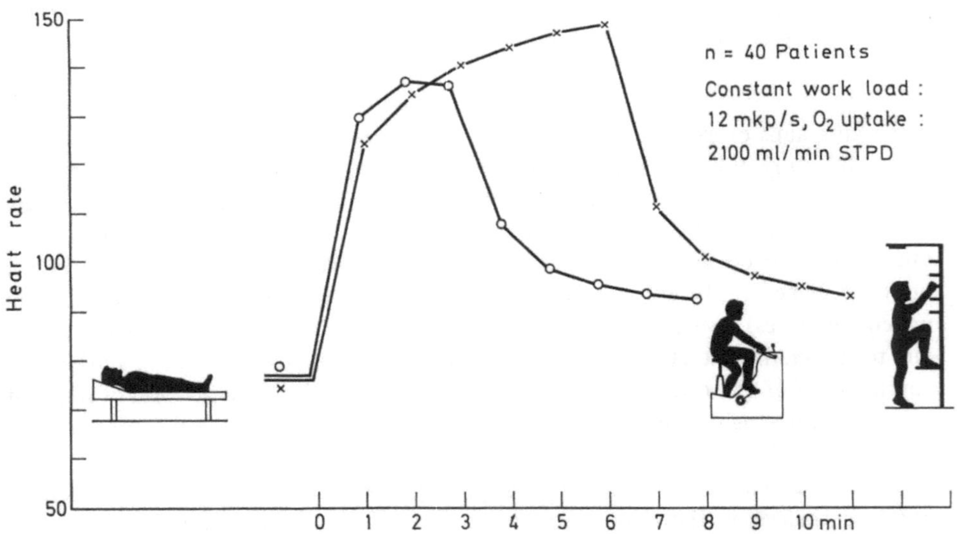

Fig. 5. Exercise testing with bicycle work in a sitting position compared to step-climbing work in supine position. At an identical work load (identical O_2 uptake during exercise), step-climbing work involving large muscle mass can be tolerated significantly longer than bicycle work. Interruption of bicycle work was, in the majority of cases, due to muscle pain

suspected or known coronary heart disease. In contrast to the United States treadmill tests were only done in a small number of institutions.

In the survey which was performed in 1978, 17 deaths were reported; this is a death rate of 1 in 42 000. Rochmis and Blackburn reported 16 deaths among a total of 170 000 tests, which is a rate of 1 in 10 000. Both figures justify the use of exercise tests as a noninvasive procedure, particularly if it serves as a method for screening patients for coronary arteriography. The fatal complication of exercise testing is about 20–80 times lower.

Among different forms of exercise an apparent difference concerning the incidence of pulmonary edema was seen. This complication occurred more often in exercise tests performed in the supine position as compared to the sitting or standing position. On the other hand, a difference in the incidence of ventricular fibrillation was not dependent on body position. The death rate was 1 in 6000 with bicycle work performed in the sitting position and 1 in 7000 with bicycle work performed in the supine position (Fig. 6). However, it was 1 in 41 000 in step-climbing work. As far as the protocol is concerned with the step test, mostly a single-stage test with submaximal or maximal load over 6 min was performed, while bicycle ergometry usually consisted of a multistage test with increasing load. The use of a short time protocol, therefore, at least with the step-climbing test, does not necessarily increase the complication rate (Fig. 7).

At the present stage some forms of exercise can be recommended for specific purposes:

1. Exercise during left heart catheterization: bicycle work in the supine position.
2. Exercise during right heart catheterization: bicycle work in the supine or semi-supine position.

	Patients n	Institutions n	Myocardial Infarct n	Pulmonary Oedema n	Dysrhythmias with defibrillation n	†	severe complications n	rate
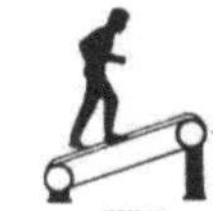	[4200	3	0	0	0	0	0	0 : 4200]
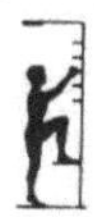	82 822	57	1	0	0	1	2	1 : 41 000
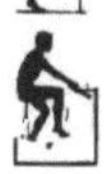	218,515	62	1	②	28	5	36	1 : 6000
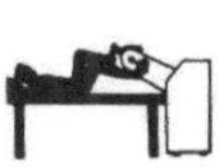	406,748	67	8	⑮	24	11	58	1 : 7500

Fig. 6. Complication rate with different forms of exercise testing. Pulmonary edema occurred more often in the supine than in the upright or sitting position. Ventricular fibrillation had a lower incidence in step-climbing work compared to bicycle work

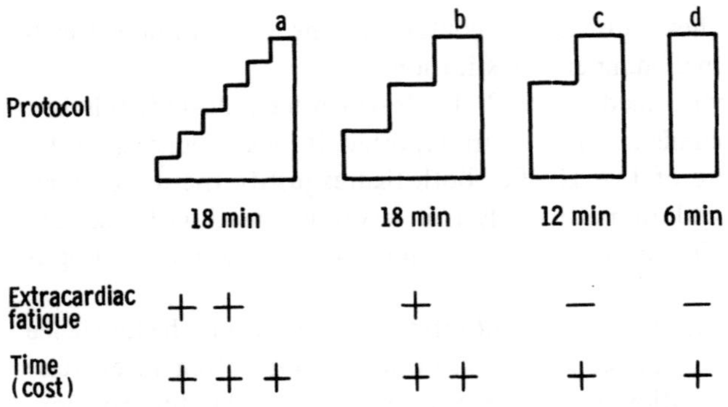

Fig. 7. Different protocols for exercise testing. Bicycle ergometry is usually done following protocol B or C, while step-climbing work is mostly performed following protocol D

3. Gated blood pool scanning during exercise: bicycle work in the supine position.
4. Early detection of myocardial ischemia in the electrocardiogram or in the thallium scan: step-climbing work or treadmill.

References

1 Davis K, Ward Kennedy J, Kemp H, Judkins MP, Gosselin J, Kilipp T (1979) Complications of coronary arteriography from collaborative study of coronary artery surgery (CASS) Circulation 59:1105–1112

2 Kaltenbach M (1976) Exercise testing of cardiac patients. Huber, Bern Stuttgart Vienna Baltimore

3 Mellerowicz H (1979) Ergometrie. Urban & Schwarzenberg, Munich Vienna Baltimore

4 Scherer D, Kaltenbach M (1979) Komplikationen ergometrischer Belastungsuntersuchungen. Dtsch Med Wochenschr 104:1161–1165

Exercise Protocol

A. Holmgren and T. Ivert

Introduction

The design of a protocol to be used in exercise testing patients with the aim of detecting ischemic heart disease should be guided by the time course of the expected development of symptoms – angina pectoris (AP) and/or dyspnea or electrocardiographic (ECG) changes.

In a study of 73 patients with ischemic heart disease investigated before bypass surgery we have shown with the aid of psychophysical scaling [4] that AP increases in intensity in a positively accelerating manner with increasing work load once a critical load has been reached (Fig. 1).

The perceived pain was rated according to a scale, shown in the following list, and the patients were carefully instructed regarding its use [5].

1. None at all
2. Extremely light
3. Very light
4. Quite light
5. Not so light, quite strong
6. Strong
7. Very strong
8. Extremely strong
9. Maximum, unbearable

We also know from a number of invasive and noninvasive measurements at rest and during exercise provoking AP that the deterioration of the pump function of the left ventricle during the development of angina attack may be a rapid event [7].

All this information indicates that the exercise protocol should be constructed so as to allow repeated measurements within a short period of time while the anginal attack develops.

The possible methods of loading patients have been reviewed repeatedly and are illustrated in Fig. 2 taken from the well-known WHO report on exercise testing (1968).

The use of a "nearly continuous increase" in load has been recommended by a large number of investigators [1, 3, 8]. Small stepwise increments in load (10–20 W) have repeatedly been found suitable for the safe provocation of myocardial ischemia and AP in a reproducible way [1].

* This work was supported by grants from the Swedish National Association against Heart and Lung Disease

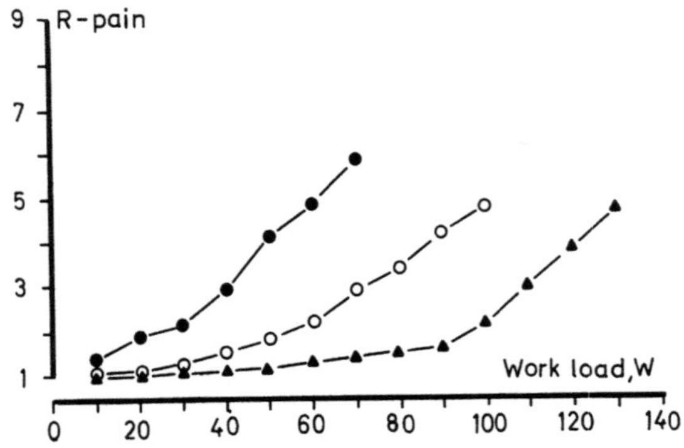

Fig. 1. Evolution of angina pectoris in 73 patients with ischemic heart disease. The patients are grouped according to work capacity. Angina pectoris was rated with psychophysical scaling, the units are arbitrary. The rated pain is scaled and there is a verbal definition of each number. Usually no unit can be given according to Borg, 1962

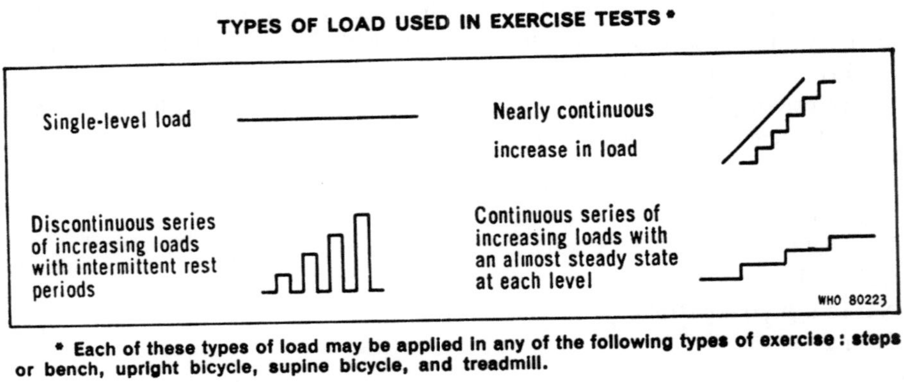

Fig. 2. WHO report on exercise tests in relation to cardiovascular function

The work can either be performed as a step test [10], walking or running on a treadmill [6], or on a bicycle ergometer [1, 3, 8]. The use of a bicycle ergometer simplifies the recording of a good quality ECG and heart rate and allows variation in body position (sitting and supine) and the addition of measurements of pressure, volume, and flow in the cardiovascular system.

Ideally it should be possible to use the same protocol in a variety of experimental situations including variation in posture, pharmacologic or other therapeutical interventions as well as when testing patients suffering from episodic chest pain or screening active asymptomatic subjects.

The following parameters should be monitored continuously or intermittently before, during, and after the work test: load (watts), slope/speed or oxygen uptake, heart rate, arterial blood pressure, and ECG. The electrocardiographic recording should ideally include 12 leads with a central terminal electrode. This necessitates averaging with the aid of a computer [2]. A compromise which has long been in use is to use six chest leads and the forehead as the position for the indifferent electrode [9]. The work test should be continued until the patient reaches a load when one or more of the following symptoms and/or signs indicate that the test should be interrupted, i.e., the end point has been reached, as is shown in the following list:

Maximal test:
1. True V_{O_2} max with flattening of the V_{O_2}-power function.
2. Symptom limited work capacity (self determined or determined by the doctor)

Submaximal test:
1. Predetermined maximal work load.
2. Predetermined maximal heart rate.
3. Predetermined maximal accepted symptom intensity and/or sign
4. Symptom-limited test (self determined or determined by the doctor).

Symptoms

1. Increasing chest pain of AP type with a highest intensity of an order that the patient onsiders would prevent him from continuing his everyday activities. The use of psychophysical scaling is recommended and helpful.
2. Severe dyspnea, especially after bypass surgery when most of the patients do not perceive pain to the same extent as before surgery.
3. Severe fatique and/or intermittent claudication.
4. Clinical signs indicating hypotension – vertigo, dizziness.
5. Physical signs of hypotension such as falling blood pressure. Severe elevation of blood pressure?
6. Electrocardiographic signs, malignant arrythmias, conduction disturbances, severe ST depressions or elevation.

Discussion

The reason for interruption of the work test and the identity of those involved should be stated explicitly. We have found psychophysical scaling of great value in evaluating the intensity of the perceived pain or dyspnea that limits the patient's ability to work on the bicycle ergometer.

It is important to stress the necessity and feasibility of adapting the protocol to the specific aim of the exercise test.

Our basic protocol is illustrated in Fig. 3. It is used in both sitting and supine exercise testing for provocation of angina in patients with known episodic pain as well as in studies screening patients for ischemic heart disease.

For special purposes we may design the protocol as is illustrated in Fig. 4, which shows the protocol used for provocation of angina in the supine position when we want to plot a function curve for the left ventricle [9]. In a similar manner we have a special protocol for studies of ejection fraction during supine exercise with isotope technique.

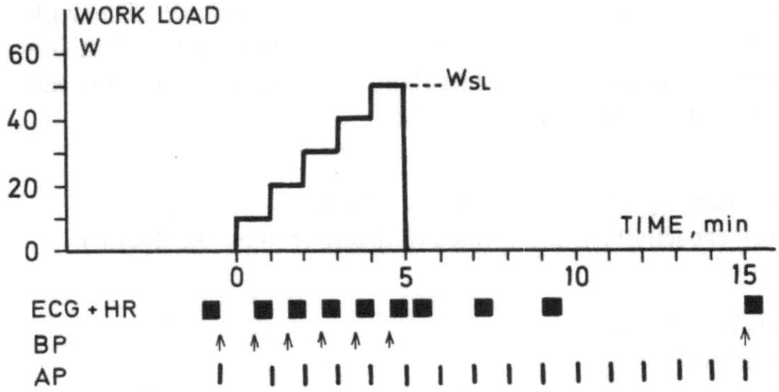

Fig. 3. Standard protocol for exercise testing patients with ischemic heart disease. W_{sl}, symptom-limited work capacity; *ECG, HR, BP,* and *AP* indicate recording of electrocardiogram, heart rate, blood pressure, and rating of angina pectoris

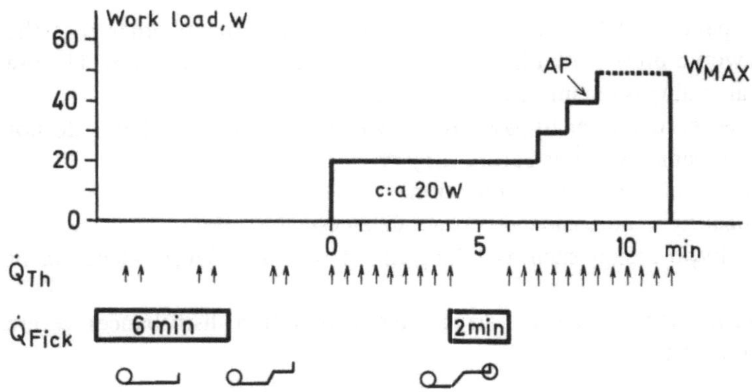

Fig. 4. Protocol for provocation of effort angina in the supine position used to plot left ventricular function curves [7]. *AP,* onset of angina pectoris. W_{max} indicates highest obtained symptom-limited work load. $\dot{Q}_{Th}$ and $\dot{Q}_{Fick}$ indicate measurement of cardiac output with thermodilution and direct Fick technique

The reproducibility one can expect in a symptom-limited, 1 min–10 W stepwise increase in exercise test is illustrated in Fig. 5. The coefficient of variation in these patients was 7.6%.

Figure 6 shows a comparison between W_{max} determined with 1-min steps and conventional 6-min steps [11]. Note that W_{max} is systematically 20 W higher and that the highest heart rate obtained is of the same order.

We have often stressed the decrease in W_{max} when patients with ischemic heart disease are exercised in the supine position. This is illustrated here with a "1' test", Fig. 7. Note that the heart rate in the supine position at symptom limitation is 13 beats lower than in the sitting position.

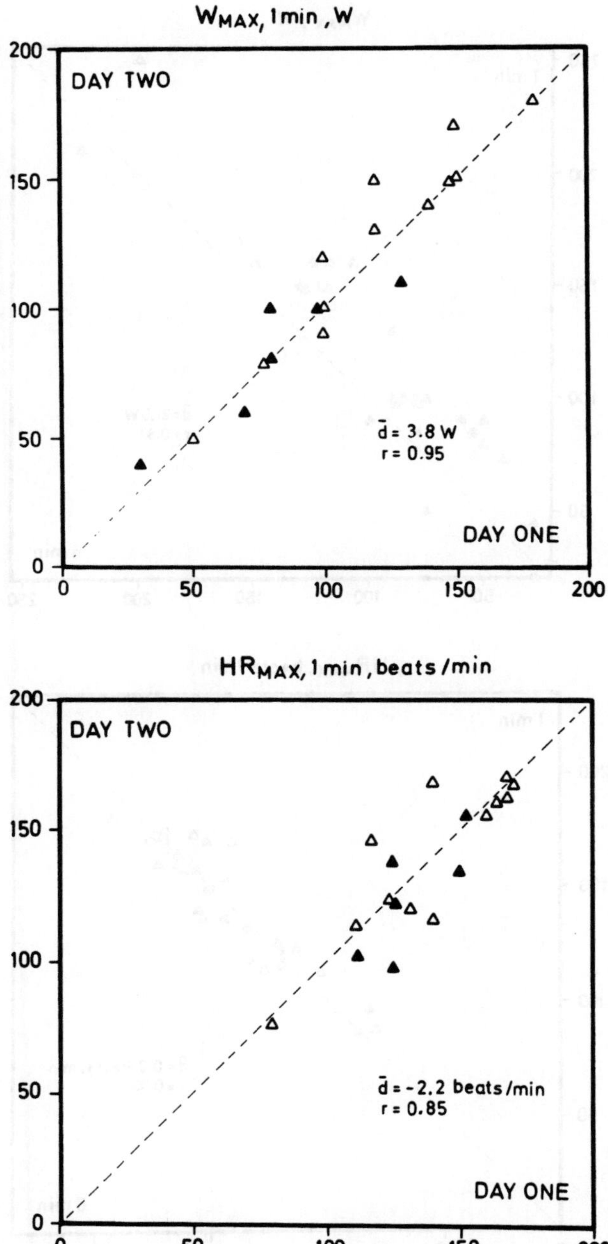

Fig. 5. Reproducibility of W_{max} and highest obtained heart rate, HR_{max} obtained with standard protocol, 10 W steps in sitting position (cf. Fig. 5) in 18 patients with ischemic heart disease on 2 separate days. *Circles* indicate women, *triangles* men. *Filled symbols* indicate patients with angina pectoris limiting the test

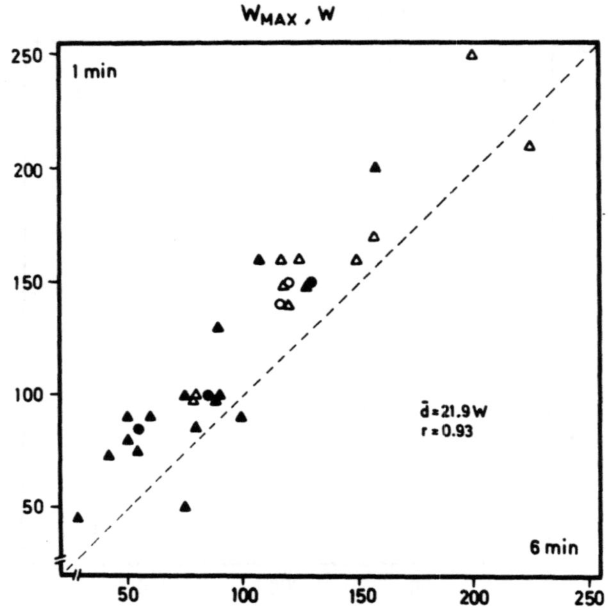

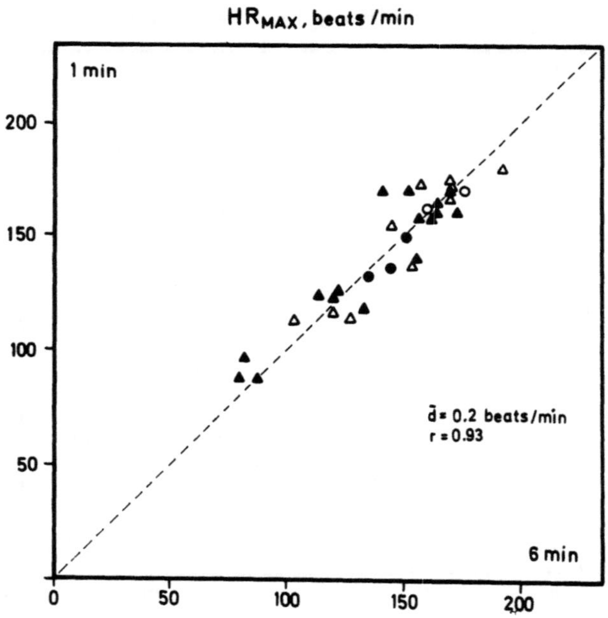

Fig. 6. W_{max} and HR_{max} in 31 patients with ischemic heart disease determined using standard protocol, cf. Fig. 5, in relation to W_{max} determined with a protocol where the patients exercise for 6 min at each work load [11]

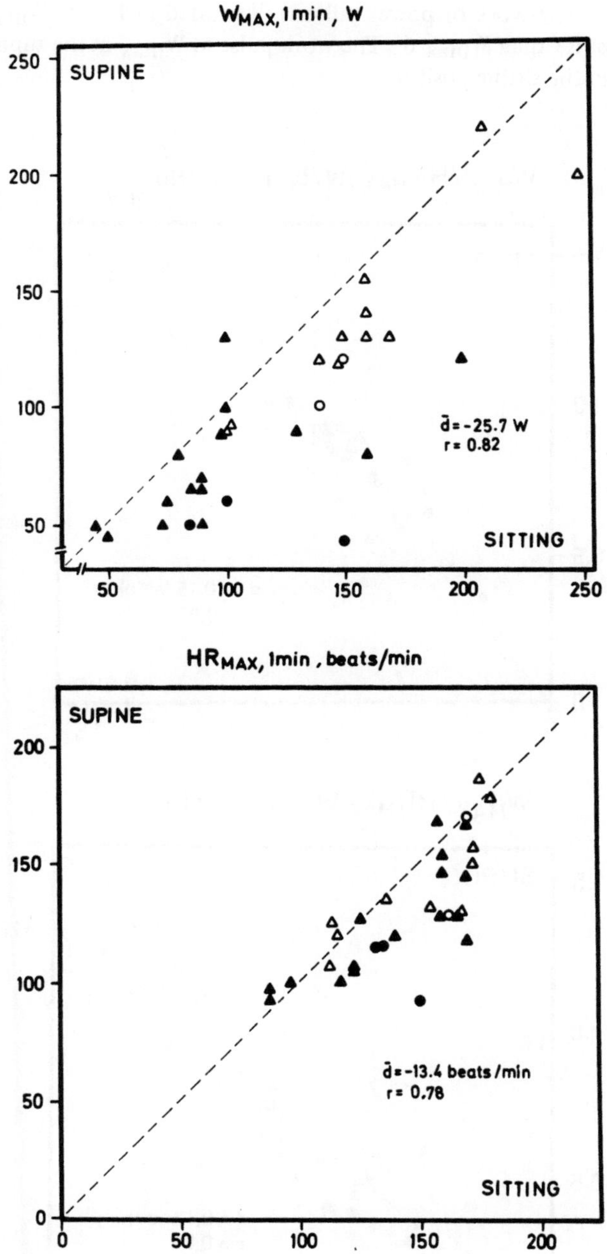

Fig. 7. W_{max} and HR_{max} determined in the sitting and supine positions, respectively, in 31 patients with ischemic heart disease. W_{max} was determined with standard protocol; cf. Fig. 3, symbols as in Fig. 5

The work or power pulse is illustrated in Fig. 8. W_{max} 1' results in a higher work pulse than W_{max} 6'. The work pulse at W_{max} in the supine position is lower than that in the sitting position.

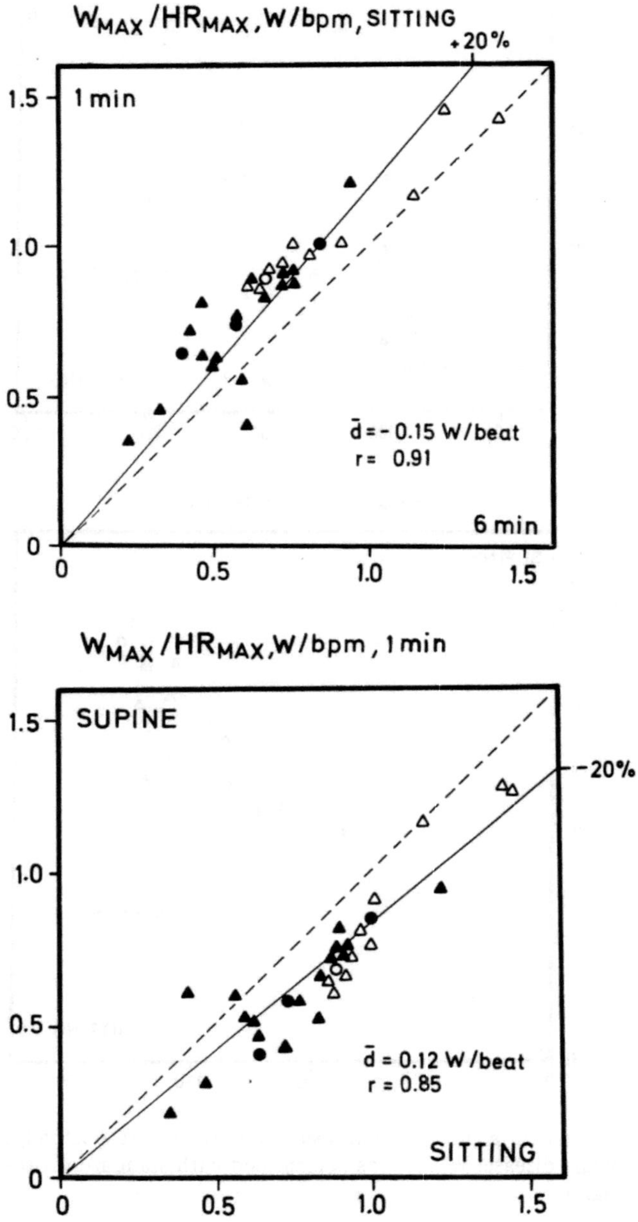

Fig. 8. Work pulse, W_{max}/HR_{max}, W/bpm, at highest work load, W_{max} in 31 patients with ischemic heart disease. *Left,* the difference between standard 1' protocol and 6' protocol. *Right,* the influence of body position. Symbols as in Fig. 5

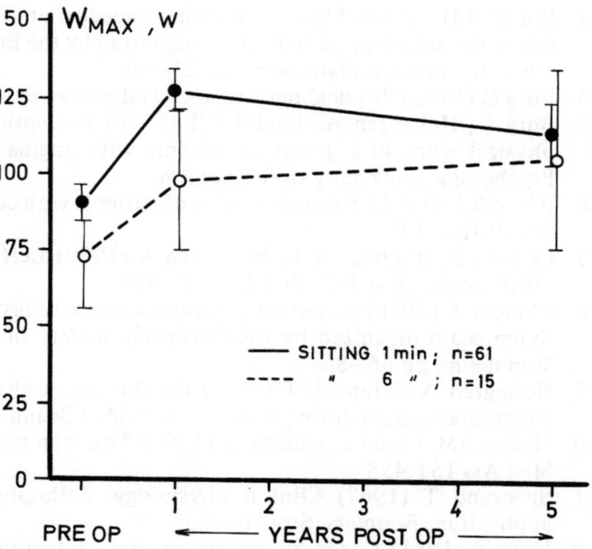

Fig. 9. W_{max} in two groups of patients with ischemic heart disease using standard 1' protocol (*full line*) and 6' protocol (*broken line*) before and after 1 and 5 years bypass surgery. Filled symbols indicate patients studied with a 1' protocol and open symbols patients studied with a 6' protocol [12]

The application of these test protocols is illustrated in Fig. 9 which shows the symptom limited work capacity before, one and five years after coronary bypass surgery.

Conclusions

We would like to stress the following:

1. Exercise protocols with a continuous or nearly continuous increase in load are well suited for testing patients with ischemic heart disease.
2. Maximal testing with symptom limitation is recommended.
3. Psychophysical scaling of symptoms is of great help, especially when repeating tests in the same individual.
4. Exercise in the supine position increases the sensitivitity of the test.

References

1 Åström H, Jonsson B (1976) Design of exercise test with special reference to heart reference to heart patients. Br Heart J 3:289–296

2 Bjurö T, Carlsson-Ejdebäck J, Schlossmann P, Varnauskas E (1978) Exercise testing in the diagnosis of coronary leasions proximal to first diagonal artery M LAD. Computers in Cardiology, 263

3 Bonjer FH (1968) Physical working capacity and energy expenditure. In: Ergometry in cardiology. Symposium organized by the European Society of Cardiology, 1967. Boehringer, Mannheim, pp 23–30
4 Borg G (1962) Physical performance and perceived exertion. Lund, Gleerup
5 Borg G, Holmgren A, Lindblad I (1979) Perception of pain in the chest during physical work in a group of patients with angina pectoris. Institute of Applied Psychology, University of Stockholm
6 Bruce RA (1971) Exercise testing of patients with coronary heart disease. Ann Clin Res 3:323–332
7 Carlens P, Hindmarch T, Holmgren A (1979) Left ventricular pump function in effort angina. Eur J Cardiol 10:475–491
8 Cherchi A (1968) A synthetic triangular exercise test. In: Ergometry in cardiology. Symposium organized by the European Society of Cardiology, 1967. Boehringer, Mannheim, pp 65–86
9 Holmgren A, Strandell T (1961) On the use of chest-head leads for recording of electrocradiogram during exercise. Acta Med Scand 169:57–62
10 Master AM, Pordy L, Chesky K (1953) Two-step exercise electrocardiogram. J Am Med Ass 151:458
11 Sjöstrand T (1967) Clinical physiology. Pathophysiological basis and practical application. Bonniers, Stockholm
12 Ivert T (1981) Coronary bypass surgery. A five year follow-up. Scand J Thorac and Cardiovasc Surg Suppl 28

The Optimal Lead System for Detection of Ischemic Myocardium

M. Niederberger and S. Panzer

Various electrocardiographic lead systems are widely used for exercise testing and no system can be called optimal for all purposes. A single thoracic bipolar lead requires little time for applying the electrodes. Furthermore, lead CM5, CC5, CB5, or CH5 has a relatively high signal to noise ratio which is especially important in persons with a high exercise capacity or during treadmill exercise. In these regards, the Frank lead system is inferior and the conventional 12 leads rank in between. However, the signal to noise ratio can be improved by computer methods, and the importance of time or cost for using the system may be weighed individually by taking other costs and the purpose of exercise testing into account, such as screening populations with a low prevalence of disease or selecting patients with probable disease for coronary angiography. In this paper, the comparison is primarily based on the diagnostic values of criteria that can be derived from the lead systems under discussion, specifically on quantitative relationships between the degree of ST segment displacement during standardized exercise testing and the probabilities of the presence or absence of reversible myocardial ischemia with respect to its location and severity.

ST segment alterations in the most commonly used bipolar chest leads, such as leads CM5 and CB5, are of similar diagnostic power. Reported values of sensitivity and specificity for significant coronary disease vary greatly, being dependent on patient selection or angiographic criteria, methods of exercise testing, and lead strength. However, in comparison to multiple lead systems a somewhat lower sensitivity of bipolar leads has been established. Two recent studies [3, 8] related bipolar lead CM5 to at least six of the conventional 12 leads, including V_3–V_6. Significant coronary artery disease was diagnosed when angiography revealed more than 70% [3] or more than 75% [8] coronary stenosis. A significant ST segment change during maximal or near maximal treadmill exercise testing was represented by an horizontal or downsloping depression of 0.1 mV or more [3, 8] or a slow upsloping depression of 0.2 mV or more [3] 80 ms after the J point.

Pooling the data from both studies shows that the multiple leads yielded 5.6% more positive results than CM5 at a specificity level of 87.4%. A relatively low sensitivity of the single unipolar chest lead V5 is in accordance with the experience that important information may be lost by using only one precordial electrode (Table 1).

Results of pooling the material from five studies [1, 2, 3, 4, 6, 8] in which the conventional leads were used during maximal or near maximal exercise are shown in Table 2. Again, as an average, the criterion of 0.1 mV ST segment depression during exercise testing yielded a sensitivity of 66% for significant coronary disease and a specificity of 87%. In contrast, when Simoons [7] applied this criterion to the Frank lead x he found a somewhat lower sensitivity visually, even by computer analysis, but

Table 1. Pooled data of Chaitman (1978) and Sketch (1978)

	CAD	Normal	Total
N	176	127	303
Lead	Sensitivity	Specificity	Index of merit (Sens. + Spec. -1)
CM5	59.7	87.4	0.47
V5	55.7	92.9	0.49
Conventional	65.3	87.4	0.53

Table 2. Comparison of conventional 12 and Frank lead systems

Lead		Sensitivity %	Specificity %	Index of merit
Conventional[a]		66	87	0.52
Frank[b]	Visual	50	94	0.44
	Computer	63	95	0.58

[a] Pooled data of Ascoop (1971), Bartel (1974), Piessens (1974), Chaitman (1978), and Sketch (1978) (504 CAD, 229 normal).
[b] Simoons [7] (52 CAD, 86 normal)

the specificity was higher. Such a difference between the conventional and the Frank leads is at least in part due to differences in lead strength: 0.1 mV represents a relatively greater ischemic change in lead x than in unipolar precordial leads such as V5 or in the bipolar leads such as CM5 or CB5. In other words, a given patient will develop smaller ST segment depressions in lead x than in these other leads. This point is illustrated in Table 3. We compared lead CB5 and lead x in 31 patients with coronary disease and exertional chest pain. All patients had one or more significant coronary stenoses, and stress thallium scintigraphy was positive for reversible myocardial ischemia. At the occurrence of chest pain during exercise testing, ST segment depression averaged 0.17 mV in lead CB5 (in terms of lead strength, CB5 is comparable to lead CM5 or V5). Simultaneously, a 30% smaller ST segment depression was measured in lead x. However, computer measurements from lead x yielded the same number of ST depressions of 0.1 mV or more as did the visual measurements from lead CB5. Therefore, the same sensitivity was achieved by both methods despite the difference in lead strength which should result in a higher specificity of measurements from lead x than from lead CB5 when a given ST voltage is used as an ischemic criterion.

The reason for improved diagnostic accuracy by computer analysis, which is indicated by the data of Simoons and by our data, is at least in part the reduction of methodological variability of measurements. The variability of ST segment measurements in our patient material (Table 3) is represented by the variation coefficients, and is only in part due to intersubject variability since the greater variability of visual measurements in lead CB5 has also been demonstrated intraindividually when the same subjects were tested several times [5]. In this study, each one of eight patients per-

Table 3. Comparison of the transthoracic bipolar lead CB5 and the Frank lead

N = 31
Coronary stenosis ⩾ 70%
Stress thallium scintigraphy positive

Lead	Sensitivity (ST ↓ ⩾ 0.1 mV)	ST ↓ (mV)	Var. coeff. (SD/M)
CB5 (Visual)[a]	74%	0.17 ± 19	109%
X (Computer)[a]	74%	0.13 ± 11	81%

[a] Immediately after SL max bicycle exercise

formed seven maximal bicycle exercise tests. The clinical condition remained stable during the period of the investigation and all tests were terminated because of chest pain. Maximal heart rates as well as maximal work loads on the bicycle ergometer were reproducible with average relative variation coefficients of 4% and 7%, respectively. Greater intraindividual variability of visual ST segment measurements in lead CB5 was indicated by greater variation coefficients (< 0.05): the mean value from eight subjects was 63%. In contrast, the respective value was only 33% for computer measurements in lead x, 75 ms after R peak (Table 4).

Summarizing the previous arguments, it seems quite well established that at a given specificity level, one bipolar lead has a 5%–6% lower sensitivity for reversible myocardial ischemia than have the 12 conventional or the Frank leads. For comparative purposes, the lead strength must be taken into account: as an example, an ST segment depression of 100 mV in lead CB5 is equivalent to approximately 75 mV in Frank lead x. The conventional leads have similar diagnostic power to the Frank leads, but they are less convenient for computer application. Use of the computer enhances the diagnostic accuracy by averaging techniques, heart rate adjusted measurements, and analysis of multiple variables. Because a combination of three bipolar chest leads performed better than one [3] and the 12 leads were superior to the single lead V5 [3, 8], it is reasonable to assume that the use of several thoracic electrodes selected for computer-aided exercise testing should further improve the detection of ischemic myocardium. In this respect, promising data have been published by Fox et al. [4]

Table 4. Intraindividual variability of ST measurements immediately after SL max bicycle exercise (each patient tested seven times)

	Patient	1	2	3	4	5	6	7	8	Mean of 8 var. coeff. (SD/M)
ST ↓ CB5	M	0.10	0.08	0.23	0.12	0.41	0.24	0.25	0.02	63%
(visual)	SD	0.07	0.02	0.14	0.05	0.08	0.13	0.06	0.02	
ST ↓ X	M	0.12	0.11	0.16	0.09	0.25	0.18	0.18	0.05	33%
(computer)	SD	0.05	0.03	0.09	0.02	0.04	0.04	0.05	0.02	

which indicate that precordial electrocardiographic mapping with 16 electrodes significantly raised the sensitivity for myocardial ischemia without a loss in specificity.

References

1 Ascoop CA, Simoons ML, Egmond WG, Bruschke AVG (1971) Exercise test, history, and serum lipid levels in patients with chest pain and normal electrocardiogram at rest; comparison to findings at coronary arteriography. Am Heart J 82:609
2 Bartel AG, Behar VS, Peter RH, Orgain ES, Kong Y (1974) Graded exercise stress tests in angiographically documented coronary artery disease. Circulation 49:348
3 Chaitman BR, Bourassa MG, Wagniart P, Corbara F, Ferguson RJ (1978) Improved efficiency of treadmill exercise testing using a multiple lead ECG system and basic hemodynamic exercise responses. Circulation 57:71–79
4 Fox KM, Selwyn AP, Shillingford JP (1979) Projection of electrocardiographic signs in praecordial maps after exercise in patients with ischaemic heart disease. Br Heart J 42:46–421
5 Niederberger M (1977) Values and limitations of exercise testing after myocardial infarction, with special reference to quantitative criteria. Acta Medica Austriaca (Suppl 9):1–46
6 Piessens J, Van Mieghem W, Kesteloot H, De Geest H (1974) Diagnostic value of clinical history, exercise testing and atrial pacing in patients with chest pain. Am J Cardiol 33:351
7 Simoons ML (1975) Criteria for interpretation of exercise electrocardiograms by digital computer
8 Sketch MH, Nair ChH, Esterbrooks DJ, Mohiuddin SM (1978) Reliability of single-lead and multiple-lead electrocardiography during and after exercise. Chest 74: 394–401

Variations in Data of Exercise Tests Due to External and Environmental Conditions

J.P. Broustet, P. Guern, J.F. Cherrier, M. Sicart, and P.M. Neuville

Introduction

Many papers in the literature attempt to appraise the prognosis value of exercise tests in terms of life expectancy, numbers of narrowed vessels, left ventricular performance in conjunction with critical value of heart rate, S-T segment depression, work tolerated, etc.

Moreover, matching placebo data with data obtained in patients serving as their own controls appears to be a proper way of appraising a new drug or to point out the best association of an anti-anginal drug in a given patient.

Thus the reproducibility of data in the same patients under different conditions must be well established and carefully checked.

During a symptom-limited exercise test, the most important parameters to be considered are (1) exercise capacity (expressed as total work performance); (2) critical or symptom-limited values for systolic blood pressure, heart rate and S-T segment depression; and (3) occurrence of chest pain. It is useful to compare S-T segment depression at the same time of the exercise test or at the same subcritical heart rate and the stage of exercise test when a prefixed heart rate is attained.

Many circumstances may induce considerable variations in these parameters and it would be impossible to discuss and comment on each of them.

Thus we arbitrarily chose to present the data observed in different conditions in normal and coronary patients. First of all, we shall deal with normals and we shall discuss the effects of the weekend, beta-blockers, and nifedipine. Thereafter we will present data relating to coronary patients with exercise-induced angina with regard to the warm-up phenomenon, variations during the same day, variations from day to day in the same patients, and variations with placebo.

All the exercise tests were done on an electrically braked cycloergometer with a protocol of 30 W, for 3 min starting with 30 W. The CM5 lead was utilized; all tests were maximal or symptom limited.

Normal Subjects

Influence of the Weekend in Normal Patients

Some years ago we attempted a prospective study to determine the possible influence of the withdrawal of nitrate vapors in 83 workers at an explosives factory.

The workers came twice to the exercise test laboratory: first on Friday at the end of the afternoon and next on the following Monday morning. At both times they performed a maximal exercise test pushed up to exhaustion. Fortunately we did not find any significant variations in S-T segment from Friday to Monday because of excellent ventilation and low grade of nitrate in the atmosphere. Thus, when comparing exercise capacity in different age groups it appeared that in the youngest group there was a decrease after the weekend (Fig. 1). Conversely, in the older patients there was an increase in physical capacity just under the limit of significance, but it was found in every patient. This could be due to intense activity in the youngest group. Soccer-games, dancing, and excessive alcohol consumption during the weekend were commonly reported by the 8- to 29-year-old age group, but not by others. Conversely, physical fatique was probably higher at the end of the week in older workmen.

Another point to be stressed was the considerable loss of exercise capacity with increasing age (Fig. 2). As most of the workers had the same type of physical activity at work, the older group is probably at a higher percentage of its $\dot{V}O_2$max and thus fatique is more important on Friday afternoon in this group.

Influence of Beta-Blockers

Atenolol at the rather high dose of 200 mg was administered 3 h before exercise tests to 11 normal medical students (mean age, 23 years) (Fig. 3). They all showed a frank decrease in systolic blood pressure, in maximal heart rate, and in heart rate at the same load, but the variations in maximal exercise capacity were different following the pre-

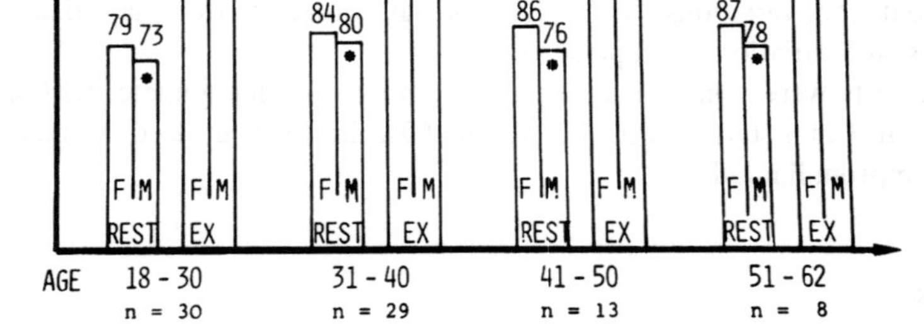

Fig. 1. Resting and maximal heart rate before and after weekend in workers exposed to nitroglycerin (N = 83). Total work (kpm/kg of body weight) performed on Friday afternoon and early on the next Monday morning. There is a trend toward a decrease in exercise capacity in the youngest group and toward an increase in the eldest group in spite of the same maximal exercise heart rate on Friday and Monday

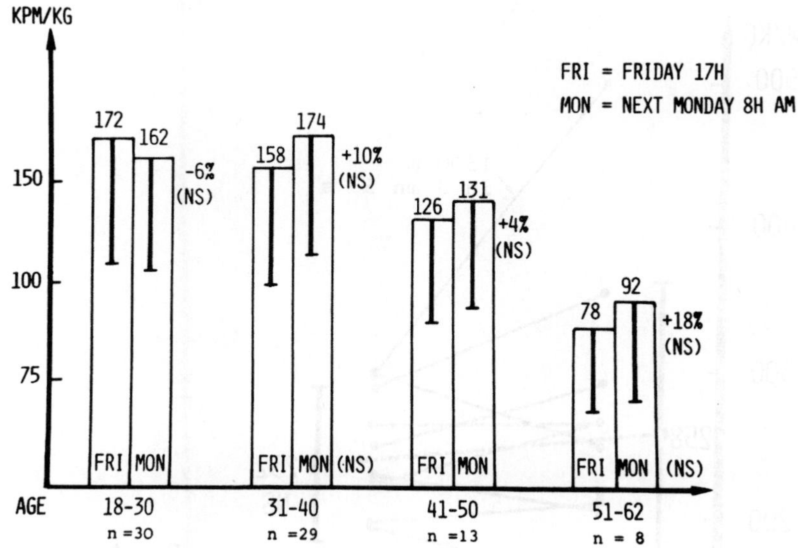

Fig. 2. Maximal work before and after weekend in workers exposed to nitroglycerin (N = 83). In spite of a significant reduction in resting heart rate, there was no change in maximal values

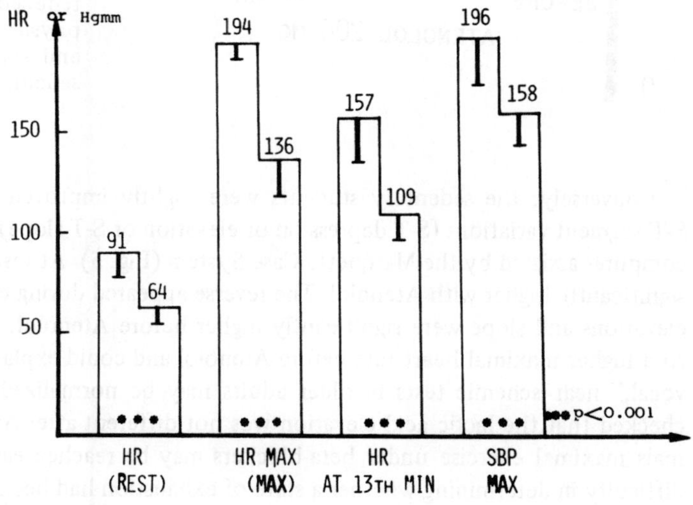

Fig. 3. Circulatory changes at maximal exercise induced by 200 mg Atenolol in 11 students. Reduction of resting heart rate (beats/min) at rest (*HR (rest)*), maximal heart rate (*HR max*), heart rate at the same submaximal level of exercise (13th min) and of systolic blood pressure at the end of exercise (*SBP max*)

vious physical fitness tests (Fig. 4). In those who were well trained Atenolol induced rather a decrease in exercise capacity, especially in the top-rank athlete who, after beta-blocker, fell from 360 W to 240 W with a maximal heart rate of 126 beats per minute instead of 186 beats per minute.

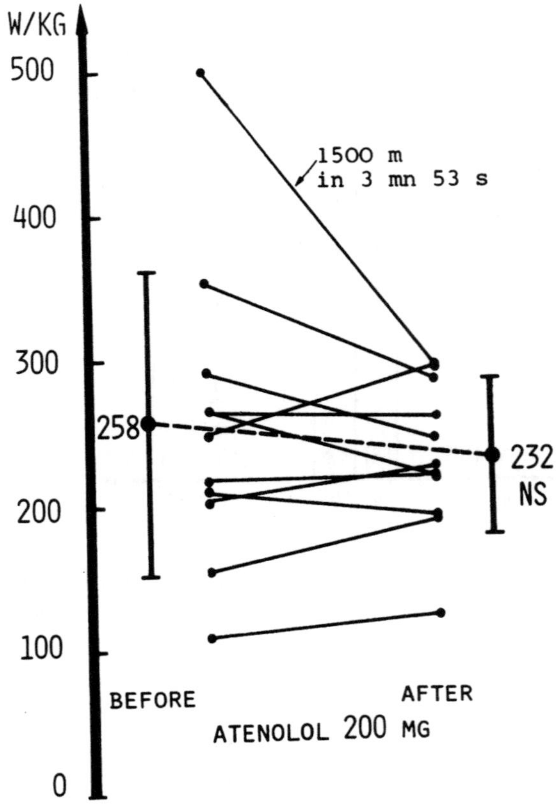

Fig. 4. Changes in maximal work in 11 normal students with Atenolol. Maximal exercise capacity (kpm/kg) was not significantly decreased in the total group, but it was reduced among the more physically trained students and slightly increased among sedentary students

Conversely, the sedentary students were slightly improved. The exercise-induced S-T segment variations (S-T depression or elevation or S-T slope) were studied with the computer assisted by the Marquette Case System (Fig. 5). At rest the S-T elevation was significantly higher with Atenolol. The reverse appeared during exercise as S-T segment elevations and slope were significantly higher before Atenolol. This was probably due to a higher maximal heart rate before Atenolol and could explain why so many "equivocal," near-ischemic tests in older adults may be normalized by beta-blockers. We checked that the lactic acid elevation was not different after Atenolol because in normals maximal exercise under beta-blockers may be reached earlier, thus leading to a difficulty in determining whether a state of exhaustion had been reached.

We used the same approach with nifedipine in 15 normal students (mean age, 27 years) (Table 1). The only different results concerned the resting heart rate and the maximal diastolic blood pressure due to large individual variations; the decrease in maximal exercise capacity was not significant, but all the participants complained of increased muscular fatique after nifedipine. There was a contrast between the slight increase in heart rate for the same load and the decrease in maximal heart rate due to the occurrence of premature muscular fatique.

It is ovious that in contrast to warm-up, phamacologic vasodilatation does not improve the exercise capacity.

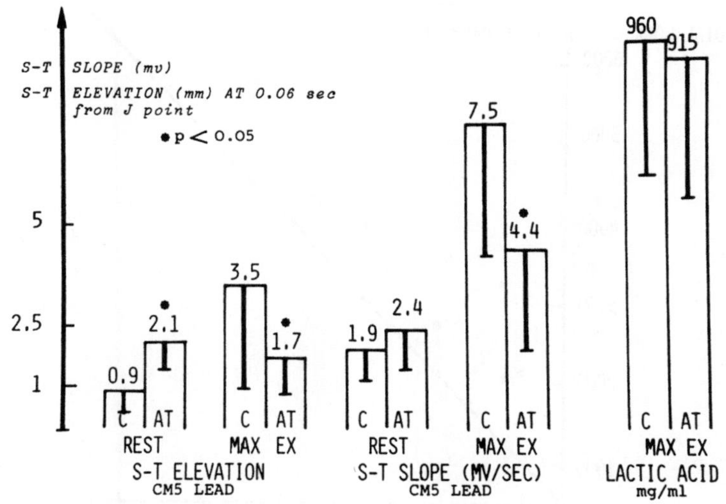

Fig. 5. Changes of S-T segment after 200 mg Atenolol (computer measurement), 11 students. Changes in *S-T elevation* and *S-T slope* at rest and at time of maximal exercise before (*C*) and after (*AT*) 200 mg Atenolol. There was no significant change in the level of lactic acid at maximal exercise

Some Causes of Variations in Coronary Patients

Warm-up Phenomenon

Sixteen patients with exercise-induced angina performed a first graded exercise test until the appearance of pain. As soon as the pain disappeared a second test was started. Thus the duration of warm-up was variable following the first exercise test as the first exercise test was itself acting as a warm-up. All patients but five improved their exercise capacity in a mean proportion of 26% ($P < 0.01$) (Fig. 6).

This progression appeared to be due to a true reduction of ischemia. At the same heart rate there was in 15 of 16 patients a decrease in S-T segment (mean, 31%) (Fig.

Table 1. Variations after 20 mg nifedipine in 15 normal students

	H rest	H 120 W	H max	SBP max	DBP max	Total work
Before nifedipine	83.40 12.58	146.00 12.07	189.73 18.81	177.00 14.37	70.00 26.19	18028.00 7073.16
After nifedipine	93.47 8.22	150.33 14.59	178.20 13.19	174.20 14.84	54.07 29.26	15810.67 6454.66
D	10.07 (+12.07%)	4.33 (- 3%)	0.93 (- 6.08%)	2.00 (- 1.6%)	17.00 (- 23%)	2217.33 (- 12.3%)
P<	0.005 N.S.	0.10 N.S.	0.40 N.S.	0.40 N.S.	0.01 N.S.	0.20 N.S.

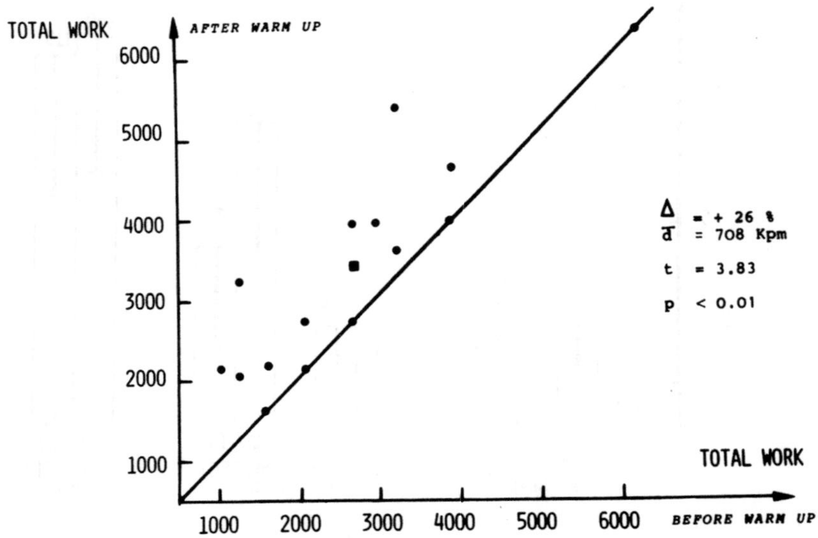

Fig. 6. Improvement of symptom-limited exercise capacity by warm-up in 16 coronary patients with severe angina

7). The second-wind phenomenon was obviously as demonstrated in Fig. 8, which depicts the S-T segment depression in CM5 lead at rest and at the same stages of exercise test in different conditions. Thus, an exercise test performed, for example, immediately after a long walk from the parking lot of the hospital may lead to the underestimation of the severity of the sublying artery disease.

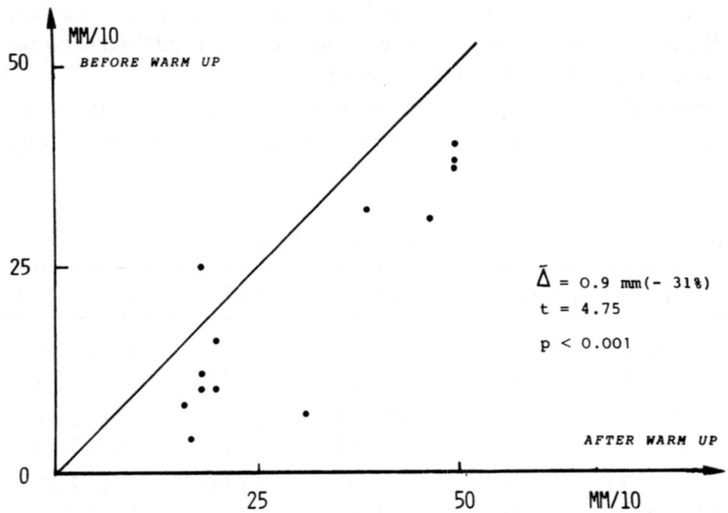

Fig. 7. Decrease of S-T segment depression at same heart rate after warm-up in 13 coronary patients

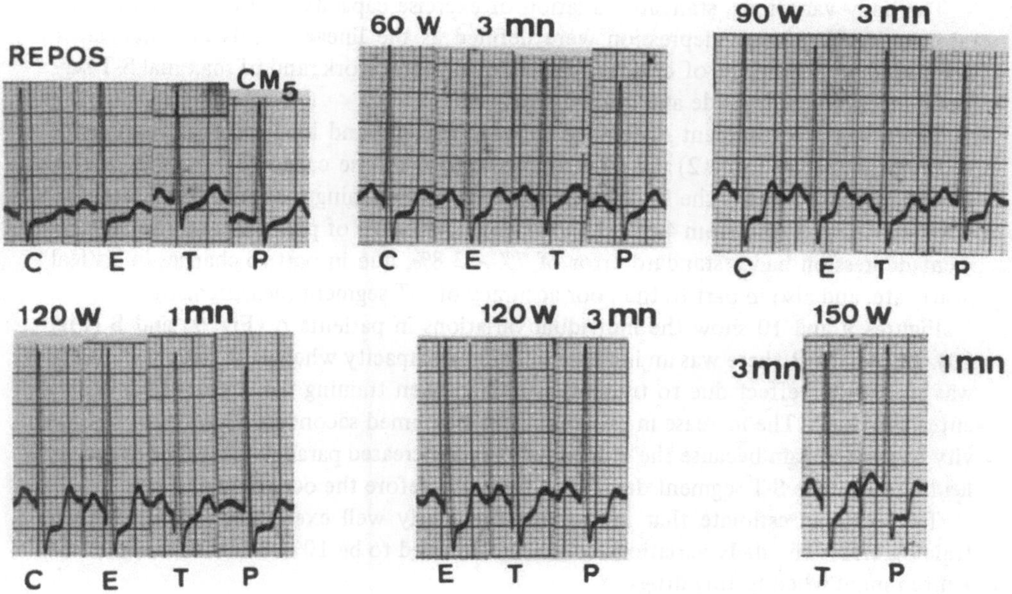

Fig. 8. Amplitude of S-T depression in different conditions. Left main trunk stenosis (80%). *C,* control test on 1st day; *E,* warm-up test started 2–3 min after the end of C; *T,* test started on day 2 or day 3 just after 0.75 mg sublingual NTG; *P,* test started on day 3 or day 2 after a placebo of T. Note the striking differences in S-T segment at the same time of exercise and the progression of exercise capacity with warm-up, placebo, and NTG

Reproducibility of Exercise Tests Throughout the Duration of Study in Coronary Patients

Patients using a common dosage of long-acting nitrates are always dramatically improved by sublingual nitroglycerin. This was such an unexpected result for the maker of this drug that he sportingly accepted a long-range contest between placebo and the drug. Four patients with exercise-induced angina, remaining within a training group for more than 4 months, carried out 40 sessions of training including first callisthenics followed by a graded exercise test. Pain was the exclusive factor for cessation of the exercise test.

Three hours before the session each patient took either placebo or durule of nitroglycerin with progressive intestinal absorption. The dosage was 2.5 mg. The randomization of allocation was different for each patient.

Finally, the patients performed 20 exercise tests with drugs and 20 with placebo at 11 p.m. between 25 January 1977 and 25 May 1977.

The daily variations, standard variation of exercise capacity, critical value of heart rate, and S-T segment depression were defined as the linear correlation coefficient between daily variations of critical heart rate and total work, and of maximal S-T segment depression amplitude and critical heart rate.

There was no significant difference between placebo and long-acting nitroglycerin.

Under placebo (Table 2) the standard error for exercise capacity was 6.4%–11.4% of the mean (9.8% for the set of four patients). Concerning maximal heart rate, the standard error ranged from 4.8%–12.9% (7.5% for the set of patients) and the S-T segment depression had a standard error of 7%–13.8%, due in part to changes in critical heart rate, and also in part to the poor accuracy of S-T segment measurement.

Figures 9 and 10 show the individual variations in patients A (Fig. 9) and B (Fig. 10). In patient B there was an increase in exercise capacity whereas in patient A, there was no further effect due to training as he had been training for 2 years in order to enter the study. The increase in exercise capacity seemed secondary to a loss of sensitivity to anginal pain because the critical heart rate increased parallel to exercise capacity, leading to a huge S-T segment depression of 6 mm before the occurrence of pain.

Thus we can estimate that in patients previously well exercised, with no further training effect the daily variations could be estimated to be 10%. These data should be kept in mind when testing drugs.

Variations Following the Time of Exercise Tests on the Same Day

When testing a new drug one aim is to determine the duration of the effect of a single dose. Thus, when we carried out an assay of Molsidomin, a potent vein dilator, we

Table 2. Standard error and mean value of exercise data during 20 exercise tests under placebo (double-blind test)

Daily data (mean and standard error)	Patients A	B	C[a]	D
Total work (KPM)	4514	7742	8302	4293
	± 459	± 459	± 950	± 490
↑ Linear correlation [r] ↓	↑ [0.44] ↓	↑ [0.44] ↓	↑ [0.60] ↓	↑ [0.39] ↓
Critical heart rate (bpm)	129	111	110	125
	± 6.2	± 5.6	± 8.6	± 5.7
↑ Linear correlation [r] ↓	↑ [0.17] ↓	↑ [0.66] ↓	↑ [0.69] ↓	↑ [0.28] ↓
Maximal S-T Depression (MM)	2.43 0.17	4.66 0.66	5.27 0.73	2.95 0.38

[a] Beta-blockers at same dose during the trial

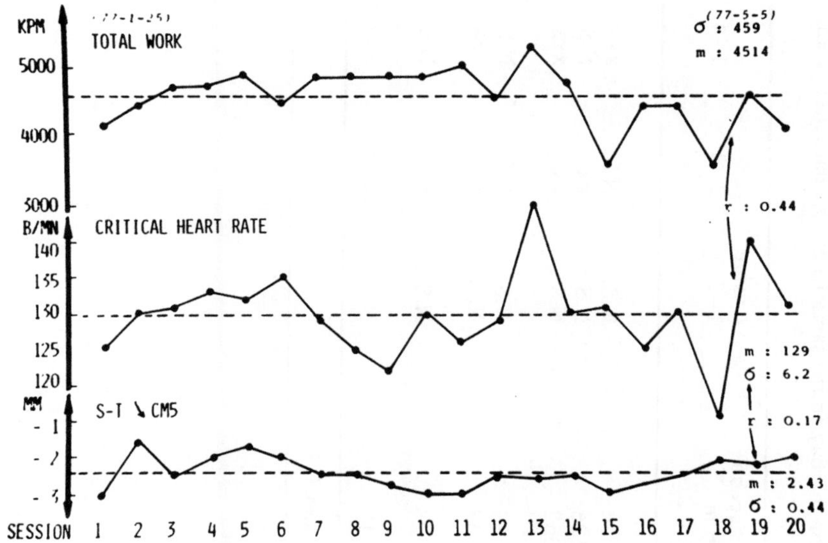

Fig. 9. Variations of exercise parameters during 20 symptom-limited exercise tests in a coronary patient (*A*) under placebo

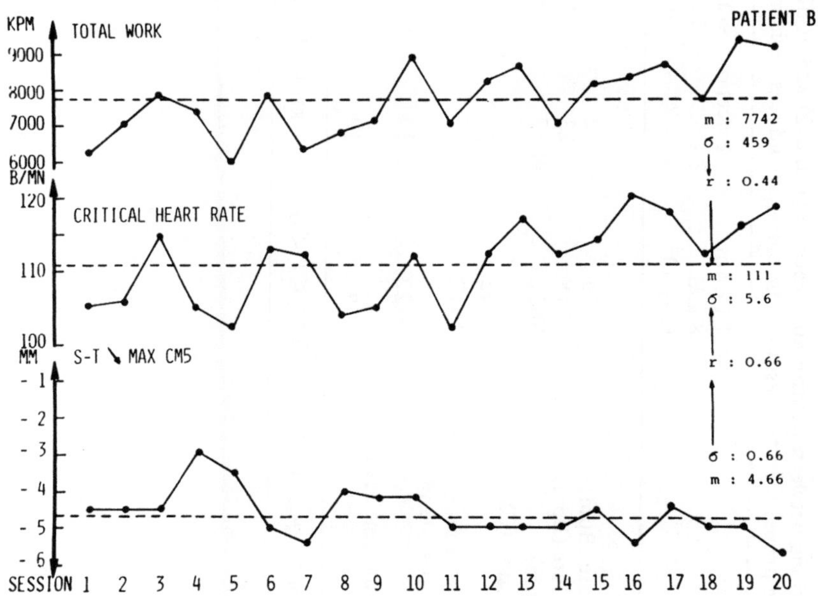

Fig. 10. Variations of critical values of work, HR, S-T ↘ with placebo progressive improvement of exercise capacity in a coronary patient

Table 3. Variations between control and placebo (1 and 2) and at different times of the day in the same 15 angina patients; 11 a.m. is obviously the proper time for best exercise capacity and least ischemia

	1 Control 8 a.m. (day 1)	2 Placebo 8 a.m. (day 2)	3 Placebo 11 a.m. (day 2)	4 Placebo 2 p.m. (day 2)	*P* value 1–2	2–3	3–4
Mean values of							
Resting heart rate (Bpm)	75	72	70	79	N.S.	N.S.	xxx
Maximal heart rate (Bpm)	118	123	126	126	N.S.	xx	N.S.
Total work (Kpm)	3632	4037	4727	4062	N.S.	xx	xxx
Max S-T depression (CM5 lead) (mm x 10)	34	35	33	34	N.S.	N.S.	N.S.
Work at same heart rate (Kpm)	1913	1955	2802	1848	N.S.	xxx	xxx
S-T depression at same FC (mm x 10)	22	19	15	24	N.S.	x	N.S.
S-T depression at same load (mm x 10)	21	18	10	17	N.S.	xxx	xxx

P values N.S. $P \geqslant 0.1$ x $0.05 \leqslant P < 0.1$ xx $0.01 \leqslant P < 0.05$ xxx $P < 0.01$

Table 4. Some pitfalls in reproducibility of exercise tests

Exercise capacity	
	Circadian rhythms?
1)	Schedule Morning psychasthenia, afternoon fatique Fasting versus postprandial state
2)	Tolerance to exercise test increasing or decreasing, motivation, fear,
3)	Interval between tests (long-term trial of drug) Changes in physical conditioning may mask a beneficial or adverse effect of drug Asymptomatic changes in coronary bed may mask a beneficial effect of drug or physical training
4)	Variations in appreciation of self-limiting pain
5)	Warm-up, external temperature, and barometric pressure
6)	Slight changes in calibration of cycloergometer
7)	Concealment of added therapy
8)	Schedule of drug administration
ECG	
Variations in	Place of leads Calibration Thorax position: bending forward or vertical

used to give at 7:30 a.m. double blind on alternate days, either the drug or the placebo, and the patients were asked to perform a symptom-limited exercise test at 8 a.m., 11 a.m., and 2 p.m. A small amount of lunch was taken at noon. On a previous day, a control test was performed with no drug or placebo to obtain a reference value versus the placebo effect.

Table 3 shows (1) a placebo effect at 8 a.m. with respect to control values, concerning exercise capacity, S-T segment depression, and critical heart rate; (2) an improvement, probably due to warm-up secondary to morning activities from 8 a.m. to 11 a.m.; and (3) the adverse effects of even a light meal on exercise capacity and circulatory response in coronary patients.

Thus, when testing the duration of activity of a single dose, placebos are absolutely mandatory for, with the drug itself, the meal will produce a decrease in performance.

Finally, there are many possible pitfalls which must be considered to insure that the data of exercise tests are reproducible and reflect the only basal circulatory and electrocardiographic responses to exercise. The causes of such shortcomings are summarized in Table 4.

Each of them should be carefully kept in mind in any trial for the appraisal of variations due to drugs, physical training, and surgery.

Indeed, the ideal patient who could repeat exactly the same test under the same conditions remains still to come!

Evaluation of ECG Changes

B. Caru, S. Pirelli, C. Candotti, G. Cattafi, A. Manzini, and M. Mangiovacchi

Introduction

The interpretation of an exercise test *must* consider its poliparametric aspect, given then to every factor at the moment of the global evaluation its particular specific weight [2, 6].

With the overall aim of having quantitative interpretation of the exercise test, we studied some parameters of exercise ECG and other factors in subjects with different levels of involvement of the coronary tree.

Our investigation involved a large sample of 200 patients divided into two groups of patients according to the coronary situation shown by coronary angiography.

Group I consisted of 100 patients, 88 males and 12 females, with a mean age of 46.75 ± 8.65 years; their coronary angiography was normal or an involvement of a single branch was present, exception done for the left anterior descending (LAD) branch.

Group II consisted of 100 patients, 96 males and 4 females with a mean age of 51.10 ± 7.26 years; these patients had a significant involvement of the three coronary branches.

None of the patients had a positive history of myocardial infarction and neither did the resting ECG shown specific signs of necrosis. All the patients performed exercise tests on a bicycle ergometer. None of the patients had digitalis treatment. When present, a beta-blocking treatment was withdrawn 7 days before the exercise test. Some data obtained using the exercise test were studied with a linear multivariate discriminant statistical analysis.

Five "independent" variables obtained using the exercise test are considered here and classified as follows: A, angina; B, entitity of ST downsloping; C, type of ST-segment; D, total work performed; E, duration of ischemia.

The variables are codified as follows: A: 1 if absent, 2 if present; B, the entity expressed in millimeters; C, 0 if the ST is normal; 1 when the ST is slowly upsloping; 2 when horizontal or downsloping; D, the total work is expressed in Kpm; E, duration of ischemia in minutes.

Results

The statistical analysis made it possible to quantify the five variables considered. For each single variable its mean value in group I compared to the value in group II was significantly different.

Then for each single variable, independent of the fact that it belonged to one of the two groups, a coefficient of the discriminating equation was calculated. This coefficient was utilized to define the degree of likelihood for an exercise test to belong to group I or II (Table 1). The sum of the products of each single variable multiplied by its coefficient of discriminating equation makes up a "qualification" index, that, according to its scalar value, defines the likelihood of belonging as a single case to group I or II, and according to the entity of that coefficient also moves the case toward more "certainly" pathologic or more "certainly" normal zones.

The zones belonging to groups I and II were singled out through the discriminant analysis performed on each of the 200 examined subjects and for everyone a qualification index was obtained. The general averages were then calculated. The discriminant analysis made it possible to define the discriminant threshold (L zero) between the two groups.

The average values of the indexes for groups I and II are respectively 0.00239 and 0.01352; the discriminating threshold (L zero) is 0.00298. Moreover, each single variable has a different specific "weight" determining the qualification index; in particular the discriminant analysis shows a significant power of pathologic value for the variables B, C, and E (Table 2).

After this first approach we continued the research taking into account patients with different levels and sites of coronary involvement. We first studied patients with

Table 1. Coefficients of the discriminating equation for each single variable

	Group I	Group II
A	1.26	1.62
B	0.69	2.41
C	0.51	1.40
D	375.07	100.83
E	0.78	3.97

Table 2. F; discriminant error and percent contribution of each single variable to discrimination – All patients –

F = 23.6	Discriminant error
$P < 0.001$	$P = 0.04$

Percent contribution of each single variable to discrimination

Variables	%
A	2.87
B	18.23
C	33.08
D	1.43
E	44.96

isolated stenosis of LAD, dividing them into two groups. Group I consisted of 36 patients with a mean age of 46.4 years, with a proximal significant stenosis of LAD. Group II consisted of 39 patients with a mean age of 48.2, with a distal significant stenosis of LAD. The qualification index for proximal stenosis is 331 and that for distal stenoses is 140; the discriminating threshold (L zero) is 223. The discriminant statistical analysis shows that $F = 4.94$; $P < 0.001$; discriminant error = 27% (Table 3).

Concerning the contribution of each single variable those classified as B, C, and E are the most important (Table 3).

The results of the statistical analysis have to be considered satisfactory in spite of the high disciminating error.

The discriminating threshold (L zero) is 223 and the mean value of the qualification index is 331 for proximal involvements and 140 for distal ones.

Then, taking into account the possible functional importance of the first diagonal, we again elaborate the data, considering as proximal those stenoses of LAD located after the first diagonal when this branch is poor [4]. In this case the statistical analysis gives $F = 3.64$; $P < 0.01$ with a discriminant error of 29%.

The specific contribution to discrimination is shown in Table 4, where the variables B and E are particularly important. The discriminant threshold (L zero) is 221 with a mean value for proximal of 346 and for distal of 154.

These results are in good agreement with those presented before and so it seems in this case, that the functional importance of the first diagonal is poor.

We also studied patients with a significant involvement of RCA, Circumflex and Circumflex plus RCA. Until now we have only preliminary data, but it is possible to say that the multivariate discriminant analysis is able to give correct weight to the changes of exercise ECG in CAD [5], and to give a significant contribution in finding the different levels of involvement of the coronary tree [1–3].

As a final comment we wish to say that from our point of view it is not completely correct to utilize as the coronary angiography a reference parameter for the exercise

Table 3. F; discriminant error and percent contribution of each single variable to discrimination – Patients with LAD involvement

$F = 4.94$	Discriminating error
$P < 0.001$	$P = 0.27$

Percent contribution of each single variable to discrimination

Variables	%
A	5.28
B	40.52
C	18.74
D	2.00
E	33.43

Table 4. F; discriminant error and percent contribution of each single variable to discrimination – Patients with LAD involvement and poor first diagonal branch

F = 3.64	Discriminating error
$P < 0.01$	$P = 029$
Percent contribution of each single variable to discrimination	
Variables	%
A	8.09
B	64.32
C	0.35
D	1.45
E	25.76

test, as is often done; we would prefer to compare the exercise test to myocardial imaging during exercise, but until now insufficient data have been available on this topic.

References

1 Caru B (1971) Valutazione dell'efficienza cardiocircolatoria (La cosiddetta riserva coronarica). Atti Corso Superiore di Aggiornamento Cardiologico, Milan
2 Cohn K, Kamm B, Feteih N, Brand R, Goldschlager N (1979) Use of treadmill score to quantify ischemic response and predict extent of coronary disease. Circulation 59:286
3 De Vita C, Ciliberto GR, Gibelli G, Caru B (1977) Contributo della prova da sforzo alla diagnostica dell'angina da sforzo stabile tipica. G Ital Cardiol 7/11:1047
4 Froelicher VF, Thompson AJ, Longo MR jr, Triebwasser JH, Lancaster MC (1976) Value of exercise testing for screening asymptomatic men for latent coronary artery disease. Prog Cardiovasc Dis 18:265
5 Redwood DR, Borer JS, Epstein ST (1976) Whiter the ST segment during exercise? Circulation 54:703
6 Selzer A, Cohn K, Goldschlager N (1978) On the interpretation of the exercise test. Circulation 58:193

The Clinical Value of Computer Assistance in the Exercise Laboratory

M.L. Simoons, R. Vinke, S. Mey, and P.G. Hugenholtz

Introduction

In recent years, computer programs have been developed to assist in the exercise laboratory. The aims of such computer systems may include (a) improvement of the ECG interpretation; (b) improved standardization of the test procedure; (c) reduction of the technical tasks of the physician and the technician who supervise the test, such as control of the ECG writer and the bicycle ergometer; and (d) generation of a report of the test. At the Thoraxcenter such a system has been in routine use since 1977 [19]. Other systems have been developed in other laboratories [1, 6–9, 11, 18]. However, most of these do not perform all tasks listed above [1, 6, 8, 11, 18].

System Design

Extensive documentation of the exercise system at the Thoraxcenter has been published [15, 17, 19], and thus only a brief summary will be presented here. Exercise is performed on a bicycle ergometer with stepwise workload increments of 10 W per minute until symptoms or near exhaustion occur. The Frank-lead corrected orthogonal ECG is recorded. The system utilizes a PDP-11/10 minicomputer with disk and special video terminal [19]. The computer "asks" all relevant data prior to the test such as age, sex, length, weight, history, ECG at rest, and indication for the test. During the test the bicycle ergometer and the ECG writer are controlled by the computer, while a complete report is generated after the test. The ECG is analyzed at 1-min intervals. A-D conversion is carried out at 250 Hz (previously 500 Hz). After location of the QRS complexes, the dominant type of beat is sought and all beats with the same waveform are averaged [15, 19]. The onset and end of QRS are located automatically and measurements are made relative to these points [15].

Selection of Measurements

In order to obtain an optimal set of measurements for interpretation of the ECG, data from four groups of male subjects were studied: 86 normal subjects, selected from a population survery [13]; 52 patients with coronary artery disease with a normal ECG at rest [12]; 49 patients with a previous antero-septal myocardial infarction [16]; and 61 patients with a previous inferior wall infarction [16]. A large series of measurements were analyzed including amplitudes of the P wave, QRS complex, and ST segment, as well as ST time integrals [11].

Table 1 presents a comparison of sensitivities of P, QRS, and ST measurements in the three groups of patients. Since some of the patients had abnormal ECGs at rest, the ECG changes from rest to maximum symptom-limited exercise are presented. Threshold values for each measurement were selected such that the specificity in the normal subjects was 90%. In comparison with the normals, patients had a lower peak heart rate [12], less augmentation of the P waves, augmentation of the R wave [2], and ST segment depression as well as ST elevation.

The P wave measurements were of little diagnostic value (Table 1). In the patients with a normal ECG at rest, the highest sensitivity was obtained by the ST depression in lead X. In the patients with previous infarctions ST elevation was observed as often as ST depression, while relative augmentation of the R wave amplitude tended to occur more frequently. It should be noted that the greatest differences with the normals were obtained in different ECG leads in the three groups of patients. Furthermore, the precise measurement points where the greatest differences were obtained varied between the groups.

The data in Table 1 indicates that ST segment changes are more sensitive than R wave changes for detection of myocardial ischemia in patients with a normal ECG at rest. In patients with a previous infarction R wave changes occur more frequently. However, it is not certain whether these ECG changes are caused by myocardial ischemia, or by the scar tissue in the myocardium [16]. Further studies are therefore needed in such patients.

In male patients with a normal ECG at rest, optimal sensitivity was obtained by a combination of two ST amplitudes, or ST amplitude and ST slope, and heart rate ([12], Table 2). More complex measurements such as ST integrals or time-normalized ST amplitudes were of no benefit.

The Probability of an Abnormal ECG Response

In clinical practice an exercise test is often reported as either normal (negative) or abnormal (positive). This dichotomy is often arbitrary and artificial. In reality the ST changes are more likely to express myocardial ischemia when they are of greater magnitude, when the ST segment is more horizontal or even downsloping, when the depression occurs earlier during exercise and persists longer in the recovery period, and when chest pain is present. A better approach would be to estimate the probability of a normal or abnormal ECG response based on ST measurements and other data such as heart rate [14] and exercise tolerance [5]. This is illustrated in Fig. 1. A further refinement may be obtained by stepwise combination through Bayesian analysis of prior and posterior probabilities [3].

Limitations of Computer Processing of Exercise ECGs

The user of a computer system for exercise ECG processing should have a basic knowledge of the hardware and software which are used. The ECG amplifiers should have

Table 1. Comparison of the diagnostic value of various ECG measurements during exercise. Data are presented of the changes in each measurement from rest to maximum exercise. For each parameter a threshold was selected which resulted in a specificity of approximately 90% in the group of 86 normals. Thus the fraction abnormal findings in the normal subjects is approximately 10%. In each group the number of patients outside this range is presented as well as the percentage of the group (between brackets). The bold figures denote the measurements with the highest sensitivity in each group of patients for, respectively, P wave changes, QRS changes, ST depression (time normalized), ST depression (fixed intervals after QRS), and ST elevation. Note that the most significant ECG changes in the 3 groups of patients occur in different leads as well as at different measurement points

		Normals	CAD	Anti-MI	Post-MI
n		86	53	49	61
↓ P	X	11 (0.13)	**19 (0.35)**	**19 (0.38)**	**26 (0.42)**
	Y	11 (0.13)	8 (0.15)	5 (0.10)	9 (0.14)
	Z	**13 (0.15)**	9 (0.16)	8 (0.16)	11 (0.18)
↑ QRS 4/8	Y	9 (0.10)	12 (0.22)	7 (0.14)	**32 (0.52)**
↑ QRS 6/8	X	11 (0.13)	**19 (0.35)**	**28 (0.57)**	10 (0.16)
	Y	10 (0.12)	16 (0.30)	3 (0.06)	20 (0.32)
	Z	9 (0.10)	10 (0.18)	4 (0.08)	16 (0.26)
↓ ST 4/8	X	9 (0.10)	21 (0.39)	4 (0.08)	21 (0.34)
	Y	9 (0.10)	12 (0.22)	5 (0.10)	2 (0.03)
	Z	9 (0.10)	10 (0.18)	24 (0.48)	3 (0.04)
↓ ST 5/8	X	9 (0.10)	**23 (0.43)**	3 (0.06)	**23 (0.37)**
	Y	9 (0.10)	13 (0.24)	6 (0.12)	2 (0.03)
	Z	9 (0.10)	8 (0.15)	**25 (0.51)**	3 (0.04)
↓ ST 70	X	9 (0.10)	34 (0.64)	9 (0.18)	**29 (0.47)**
	Y	13 (0.15)	17 (0.32)	5 (0.10)	4 (0.06)
	Z	9 (0.10)	3 (0.05)	10 (0.20)	3 (0.04)
↓ ST 90	X	9 (0.10)	**37 (0.69)**	**11 (0.22)**	38 (0.45)
↑ ST 4/8	X	9 (0.10)	3 (0.05)	**20 (0.40)**	4 (0.06)
	Y	10 (0.12)	7 (0.13)	7 (0.14)	**30 (0.49)**
	Z	9 (0.10)	**10 (0.18)**	3 (0.06)	15 (0.24)

CAD, patients with coronary artery disease and normal ECG at rest; Anti-MI, patients with a previous anteroseptal infarction; Post-MI, patients with a previous posterior or inferior wall infarction

Table 2. Results of visual interpretation (0.1 mV horizontal ST depression) and of quantitative analysis of the exercise ECG in a training group of 86 normal subjects and 52 patients with coronary artery disease and in a test group of 43 normals and 43 patients. All patients had a normal ECG at rest. The quantitative ST measurements were adjusted for the normal heart rate-dependent ECG changes (HR); see [14]

	Training group		Test group	
	Sensitivity	Specificity	Sensitivity	Specificity
Visual ST ↓	0.05	0.94	0.51	0.95
ST 60_X (HR)	0.81	0.93	0.70	0.93
ST 20_X, ST 80_X (HR)	0.85	0.91	0.84	0.88

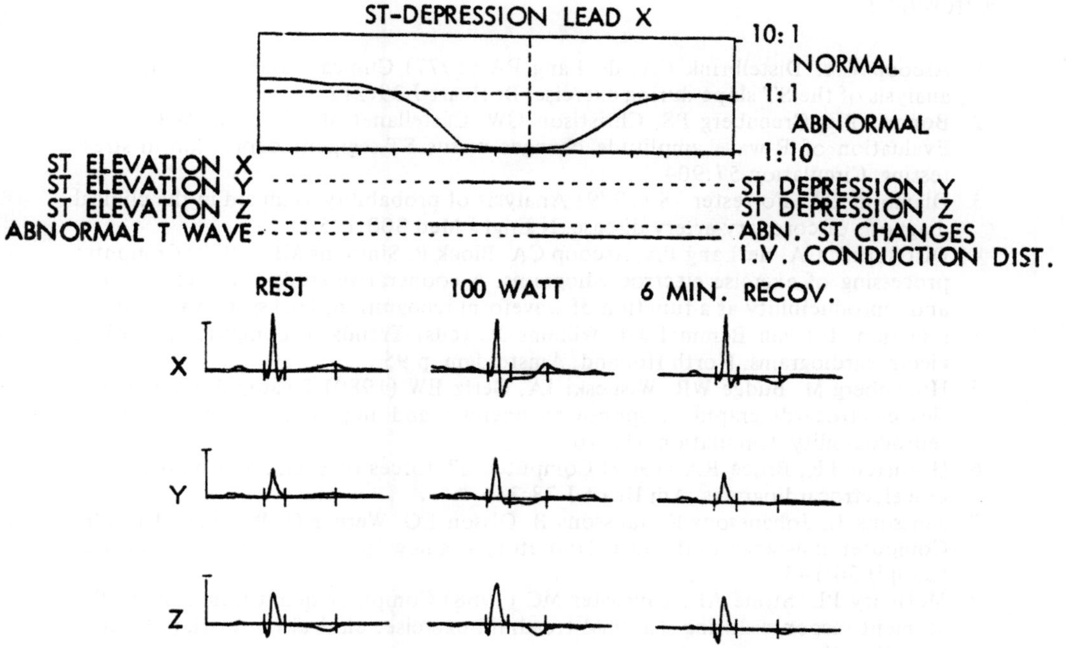

Fig. 1. Part of the printout of the report of an exercise test as generated by the computer program at the Thoraxcenter. At the bottom representative averaged complexes are presented, lead X, Y, Z of the Frank system, at rest, at peak exercise (100 W) and at the end of the recovery period. Markers indicate the onset and the end of QRS and the spatial maximum of T as detected by the computer program.

In the upper panel the graph represents the probability of a normal- or abnormal ST segment in lead X, measured at 1-min intervals. The vertical dotted line corresponds to peak exercise. Note a normal ST segment at rest and during the first 4 min of the test and a gradual development of an abnormal ST segment at higher workloads. In the recovery period the measurements return to the normal range. In the mid panel the appearance of ST depression in lead Y during two minutes before peak exercise is indicated, as well as the occurence of abnormal changes in the spatial ST vectors, and of an abnormal T wave in the recovery period

adequate frequency response. Analog digital conversion should be done at 250 Hz or greater. Furthermore, the user should realize that the measurements depend on the methods which are used for signal conditioning, such as averaging, as well as on the waveform analysis program. In particular, considerable differences may be present in the end of QRS as detected by different programs [4]. Finally, special criterial should be developed for each ECG lead system [20].

A future user should ask the manufacturer of any commercially available system for extensive documentation including the results of clinical evaluation of the system as a whole in a series of patients with independent documentation of the presence or absence of disease [10, 21].

References

1 Ascoop CA, Distelbrink CA, de Lang PA (1977) Clinical value of quantitative analysis of the ST slope during exercise. Br Heart J 39:212
2 Bonoris PE, Greenberg PS, Christison GW, Castellanet MJ, Ellestad MH (1978) Evaluation of R-wave amplitude changes versus ST-segment depression in stress testing. Circulation 57:904
3 Diamond GA, Forrester JS (1979) Analysis of probability as an aid in the clinical diagnosis of coronary-artery disease. N Engl J Med 300:1350
4 Distelbrink CA, de Lang PA, Ascoop CA, Block P, Simoons ML (1977) Computer processing of exercise electrocardiograms. A cooperative study. IV: Performance and reproducibility as a function of waveform recognition, lead system and patient selection. In: van Bemmel JH, Willems JC (eds) Trends in computer processed electrocardiograms. North Holland, Amsterdam, p 95
5 Hollenberg M, Budge WR, Wisneski JA, Gertz EW (1980) Treadmill score quantifies electrocardiographic response to exercise and improves test accuracy and reproducibility. Circulation 61:276
6 Hornsten TR, Bruce RA (1969) Computed ST forces of Frank and bipolar exercise electrocardiograms. Am Heart J 78:346
7 Janssons L, Johanssons K, Janssons B, Olsson LG, Werner O, Westling H (1976) Computer assistance in the ECG laboratory – a new look. Scand J Clin Lab Invest (Suppl) 36:145
8 McHenry PL, Stone AE, Lancaster MC (1968) Computer quantitation of the ST-segment response during maximal treadmill exercise: clinical correlation. Circulation 38:691
9 Mortara DW (1977) A new pattern recognition approach to exercise analysis. In: van Bemmel JH, Willems JC (eds) Trends in computer processed electrocardiograms. North Holland, Amsterdam, p 407
10 Pipberger HV, Cornfield J (1973) What ECG computer program to choose for clinical application – the need for consumer protection. Circulation 47:918
11 Sheffield LT, Holt JH, Lester FM, Conroy DV, Reeves TJ (1969) On-line analysis of the exercise electrocardiogram. Circulation 40:935
12 Simoons ML (1977) Optimal measurements for detection of coronary artery disease by exercise echocardiography. Comput Biomed Res 10:483
13 Simoons ML, Hugenholtz PG (1975) Gradual changes of ECG waveform during and after exercise in normal subjects. Circulation 52:570
14 Simoons ML, Hugenholtz PG (1977) Estimation of the probability of exercise induced ischemia by quantitative ECG analysis. Circulation 56:552
15 Simoons ML, Boom HBK, Smallenburg E (1975) On-line processing of orthogonal exercise electrocardiograms. Comput Biomed Res 8:105
16 Simoons ML, van den Brand M, Hugenholtz PG (1977) Quantitative analysis of exercise electrocardiograms and left ventricular angiograms in patients with abnormal QRS complexes at rest. Circulation 55:55
17 Simoons ML, Vinke R, Krebbers Th (1978) Reproducibility of computer processed exercise electrocardiograms. Comput Cardiol, p 259
18 Sketch MH, Hain CK, Esterbrooks D, Mohiuddin S (1977) Clinical experience with automated exercise ECG analysis. Comput Cardiol, p 337
19 Vinke RVM, Engelse WAH, Hoaghout T, Mey S, Simoons ML, Top P, Zeelenberg C (1977) Implementation and clinical evaluation of computer assisted analysis of exercise ECG. Comput Cardiol, p 345
20 Wolthuis RA, Froehlicher VF, Hopkirk A, Fischer JR, Kreiser N (1979) Normal electrocardiographic waveform characteristics during treadmill exercise testing. Circulation 60:1028
21 Simoons ML, Hugenholtz PG, Ascoop CA, Distelbrink CA, Land PA de, Vinke RVM (1980) Quantitation of exercise electrocardiography. Circulation 63:471

The Value of Holter Monitoring for Detection of Ischemic Heart Disease

M.L. Simoons, T. Boehmer, J. Roelandt, and J. Pool*

Introduction

The diagnosis of stable coronary artery disease can be established by making a careful history of the patient, documentation of ECG changes during episodes of coronary insufficiency, visualization of regions with temporarily impaired uptake of thallium-201 or other isotopes, measurement of impaired left ventricular function during ischemic episodes and, finally, coronary arteriography. Optimal results will be obtained when the proper methods are selected for each individual patient.

Characteristic ECG changes can be elicited through an exercise test. Furthermore, ECG changes during spontaneous ischemic episodes can be recorded by Holter electrocardiography. In this paper the relative values of these two methods will be discussed.

Holter Electrocardiography

With a small, portable tape recorder the ECG can be recorded during various activities of a patient at home, in his work or elsewhere. The ECG can be analyzed at high speed (30, 60, or 120 x normal speed) by a trained technician. With this method arrhythmias can be detected, as well as transient QRS or ST changes. For the latter purpose it is mandatory that both the recording system and the analyzer have a proper frequency response, especially in the low frequency range of the ECG. A calibration system is necessary. The patient is requested to keep a diary of his activities and complaints, if any.

A trend plot of heart rate and ST amplitude can be generated by most systems. Episodes with possible ST changes can then be marked and the ECG at those instances is recorded on paper for visual inspection.

Advantages of Holter Electrocardiography

1. ECG is recorded during normal activities. The method is particularly suited to detecting abnormalities related to specific activities, e.g., during work, and abnormalities which occur predominantly at rest.
2. No personnel is required during the recording period.
3. Holter ECG is the most sensitive method for detection of arrythmias.

---

* With technical assistance by Angela Peterse, Flora ten Cate, and Hanneke van Meurs

Limitations of Holter Electrocardiography

1. ECG recording is limited to one or two leads.
2. The occurrence of abnormalities may depend on the activities of a patient. It is not safe to instruct the patient to stress himself without supervision.
3. The sensitivity of Holter electrocardiography for detection of coronary artery disease is lower than exercise testing (see below).

Exercise Testing

Patients can be exercised on either a treadmill or a bicycle ergometer. The workload is increased gradually, e.g., 10 W/min, until the patient develops complaints or until severe abnormalities occur. The ECG is continuously displayed and recorded at regular intervals.

Advantages of Exercise Testing

1. In addition to the ECG, other information can easily be obtained during an exercise test: the physical work capacity, the patterns of the heart rate and blood pressure response, and the development of complaints or symptoms.
2. It is reasonably safe to exercise a patient under medical supervision until symptoms appear.
3. Multiple ECG leads can be obtained simultaneously, including the standard 12 leads and orthogonal leads (vectorcardiogram).

Limitations of Exercise Testing

1. The test should be attended by personel trained in interpretation of the complaints and of the electrocardiogram as well as in cardiopulmonary resuscitation. In most instances this should be a physician.
2. It is not easy to relate the workload during the exercise test to the level of other activities of a patient.

Detection of Arrhythmias

In Table 1, ventricular arrhythmias are presented in 141 patients with coronary artery disease who underwent Holter ECG and an exercise test at the Thoraxcenter. In 57 of 141 patients the same arrhythmias were observed in both tests. Eight patients had more severe arrhythmias during exercise and 76 had the highest degree of arrhythmias in the Holter ECG. These data are consistent with earlier publications as illustrated in Table 2 [4]. The greater yield of arrhythmias with Holter monitoring is probably due to the duration of the recording: 24 h in comparison with 30 min duration of an exercise test.

Table 1. Distribution of the highest grade of ventricular arrhythmias in 141 patients during Holter monitoring and during symptom-limited exercise test. (Grade 0–4 modified after Ryan et al.)

	Exercise 0	1	2	3	4	
H	22	2				0: No PVC
O	26	12		3	2	1: PVC < 5/min
L	3	1	3			2: PVC ⩾ 5/min
T	9	10	3	3	1	3: Multiform
E	11	5	5	3	17	4: Repetitive
R						
						N = 141

Detection of Repolarization Changes

The relative sensitivities of Holter ECG and exercise electrocardiography for detection of ST-T segment changes were compared in 45 patients with a history of angina pectoris. The Holter system (Oxford Instruments, Medilog II) was attached before the exercise test. Recording continued until 24 h later. Lead MC_5 was used for analysis of the ST changes.

Trend plots were generated of heart rate and the ST amplitude, approximately 60 ms after the end of QRS; ECG strips were made in all instances where ST changes were suspected in the trend recording, at points when the patient reported chest pain or other complaints, and once every hour.

Of 45 patients, 20 had no ST changes either during exercise or during 24-h monitoring. Seventeen patients had ST changes exceeding 0.1 mV in both tests, and the remaining eight patients had ST depression during exercise only (Table 3). In 13 of 17 patients with ST changes in both tests, those during exercise were of greater magnitude (Table 4), while one patient had the greatest ST changes the evening after the exercise test. This particular patient developed a myocardial infarction after an automobile accident at that time. He recovered afterward.

The greater yield of ST segment depression during exercise compared with Holter monitoring may be due to differences in the level of physical stress. The peak heart rate during exercise exceeded the highest heart rate during other activities in 41 of 45 patients (Fig. 1).

In our study we did not observe patients with ST changes during Holter monitoring and a normal exercise ECG. This is at variance with results from other centers (Table 3). This difference may be due to patient selection or to insufficient workload during the exercise tests.

Table 2. Comparison of the occurrence of the highest grade of ventricular arrhythmias in 100 patients reported by Ryan et al. [2] and in the 141 patients from the Thoraxcenter

	No PVC	Same	Most complex PVC Holter	Most complex PVC Exercise
Ryan et al. [4]	10	20	60	10
Thorax	22	35	76	8
n = 241	32 13%	55 23%	136 56%	18 7%

Table 3. Occurrence of ST segment depression or ST elevation (0.1 mV ór greater) in four studies

	No ST	Both	Holter	Exercise
Wolf [7]	23	13	5	6
Stern [6]	20	23	2	3
O'Rourke [3]	18	21	7	10
Thorax	20	17	–	8
n = 206	81 39%	84 41%	14 7%	27 13%

Table 4. ST segment changes during exercise, in comparison with Holter ECG (in millimetres = 0.1 mV)

	Exercise	0	1	2	3	4
HOLTER	4					
	3			1[a]		
	2			1		5
	1		2	3	5	
	0	20	3	4	1	

[a] Patient with myocardial infarction during Holter recording

Conclusions

Holter monitoring is the most sensitive method for detection of arrhythmias; exercise testing may give additional information, in particular when the history of the patient suggests exercise-related arrhythmias.

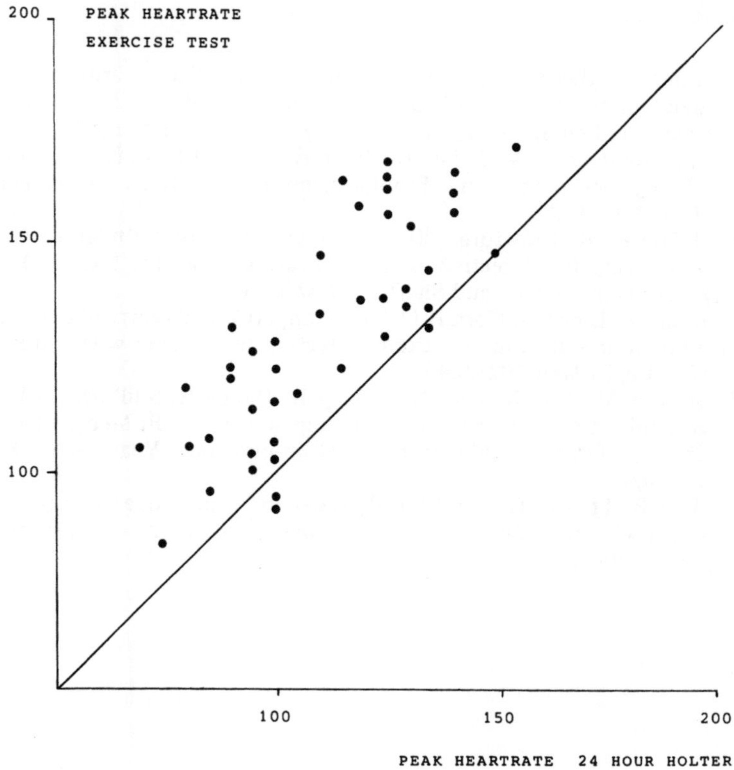

Fig. 1. Peak heart rate during 24-h Holter monitoring and during a symptom-limited exercise test in 45 patients. The line of identity is shown. Note higher heart rate during the stress test in 41 of 45 patients

On the other hand, exercise testing is the method of choice for detection of ECG changes related to myocardial ischemia. Holter electrocardiography may be used for the analysis of symptoms which are unrelated to exercise or which occur during specific activities, e.g., at work. It is mandatory that both the recording system and the playback unit have an adequate frequency response for proper representation of the QRS complex, and the ST segment [1, 2].

The method for analysis of arrhythmias differ from those for ST segment analysis. Furthermore, false negative findings obtained with Holter ST analysis may be due to the selection of ECG leads which have been recorded [5].

References

1 American Heart Association Committee on Electrocardiography (1975) Recommendations for standardization of leads and of specifications for instruments in electrocardiography and vectorcardiography. Circulation.52:11

2 Balasubramanian V, Lahiri A, Green HL, Stott FD, Raferty EB (1980) Ambulatory ST segment monitoring. Problems, pitfalls, solutions and clinical application. Br Heart J 44:419

3 O'Rourke R, Crawford MH (1978) The value of ambulatory electrocardiographic monitoring for detection ischemic heart disease. In: Mason DT (ed) Advances in heart disease. Green and Shaffon, New York

4 Ryan M, Lown B. Horn H (1975) Comparison of ventricular ectopic activity during 24-hour monitoring and exercise testing in patients with coronary heart disease. New Engl J Med 292:224–29

5 Selwyn AP, Fox K, Eves M, Oakley D, Dargie H, Shillingford J (1978) Myocardial ischemia in patients with frequent angina pectoris. Br Med J 1191–96

6 Stern S (1978) Ambulatory ECG monitoring. Year Book Medical Publishers, Chicago

7 Wolf E, Tzivoni D, Stern S (1974) Comparison of exercise tests and 24-hour ambulatory electrocardiographic monitoring in detection of ST-T changes. Br Heart J 36:93–95

Telemetry

K. Bachmann, G. Raab, and R. Zerzawy

Introduction

Since the days of Einthoven ECG telemetry has advanced so far that it is no longer just a technically fascinating method in the experimental state but is routinely used in different forms. If one defines telemetry as a method of measurement independent of the laboratory then at the present state of the art, tape recording are available (Fig. 1). In order to provide a more complex telemetry of the cardiovascular system than that provided by ECG telemetry alone, radiotelemetry of direct blood pressure measurements in the arterial system and the pumonary artery was developed in our laboratory in 1967 [1].

Telemetry of the cardiovascular system supplements standard exercise testing in the laboratory inasmuch as it gives the information on every day hemodynamic stress and the cardiovascular response to it. Up to 1978 we have studied a total of 1920 subjects with catheters in the aorta and the pulmonary artery, outside the hospital, without experiencing any complication [2]. Radiotransmission of cardiovascular parameters provides, as compared to tape and solid state recording, the possibility of continuously monitoring the patient on a scope. Therefore it is at the moment technically the only telemetric method to extend invasive methods commonly used in exercise stress testing to daily life situations (Fig. 2). Radiomonitoring gives an insight into hemodynamic stress, ectopic activity, myocardial ischemia, preload, afterload, and cardiac performance – and by calculating systolic pressure rate product – on myocardial oxygen demand even in severly ill cardiac patients during their daily life activities.

ECG Telemetry

Tape Recording and Radiotelemetry Versus Standard Exercise Testing

To evaluate ECG telemetry in the form of radiotelemetry and tape recording in comparison with standard testing we have studied 69 patients aged 35 to 70 years with a mean age of 52 years with angiographically severe multiple vessel disease. During the standard exercise testing on the bicycle in the sitting position and a 4-h radiotelemetry in the terrain, blood pressure was measured radiotelemetrically in the arterial system and in the pulmonary artery to get information about heart rate, preload, and afterload when comparing the two rate pressure product methods.

In detecting myocardial ischemia in this selected group of patients with multiple vessel disease, exercise testing is highly sensitive as compared to radiotelemetry and

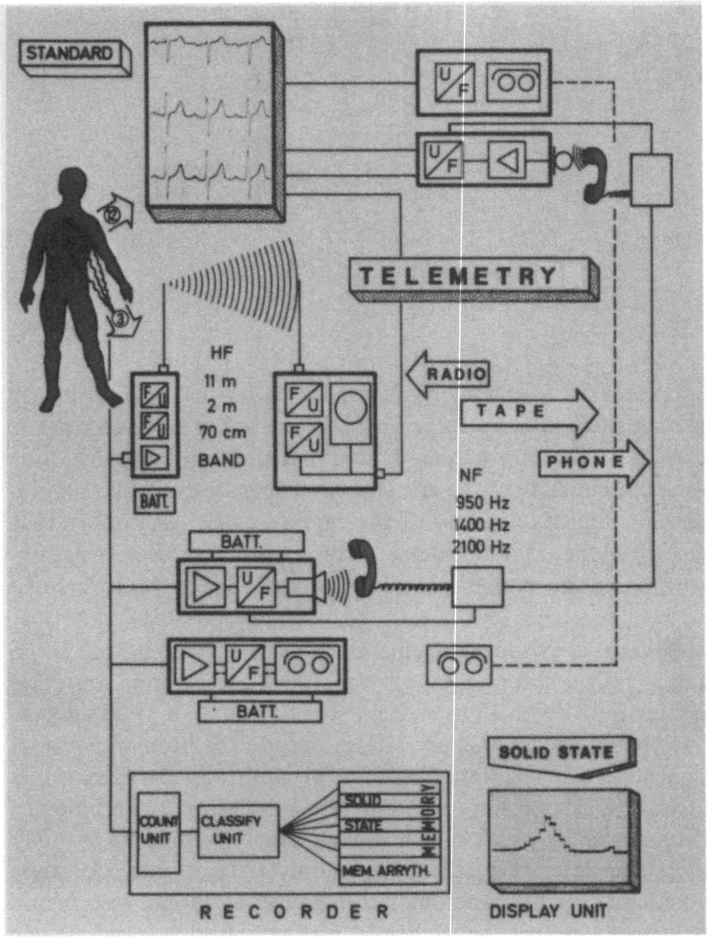

Fig. 1. Methods of laboratory remote electrocardiography: radio and phone transmission, tape and solid state recording

tape recording. It reveals ST segment depression of 0.1 mm or more in 84% of the cases as compared to 49% during radiomonitoring in the terrain (Fig. 3). In a subgroup of 29 patients in whom we studied all three methods the findings are the same. Direct tape recording with the Medilog I (Oxford Co.) is shown to be less sensitive as compared to exercise testing and radiotelemetry, demonstrating ST segment depression in 31% only. While detection of myocardial ischemia correlates with the intensity of hemodynamic stress it is remarkable that there are no statistically significant differences in exercise testing and radiotelemetry in the terrain as far as pulmonary artery pressure, arterial pressure, and pressure rate product are concerned, but nevertheless, a 4-h radiotelemetry monitoring has only 58% of the sensitivitity of exercise testing in detecting myocardial ischemia. This discrepancy may therefore be explained by the longer duration of submaximal workload during standard exercise testing and techni-

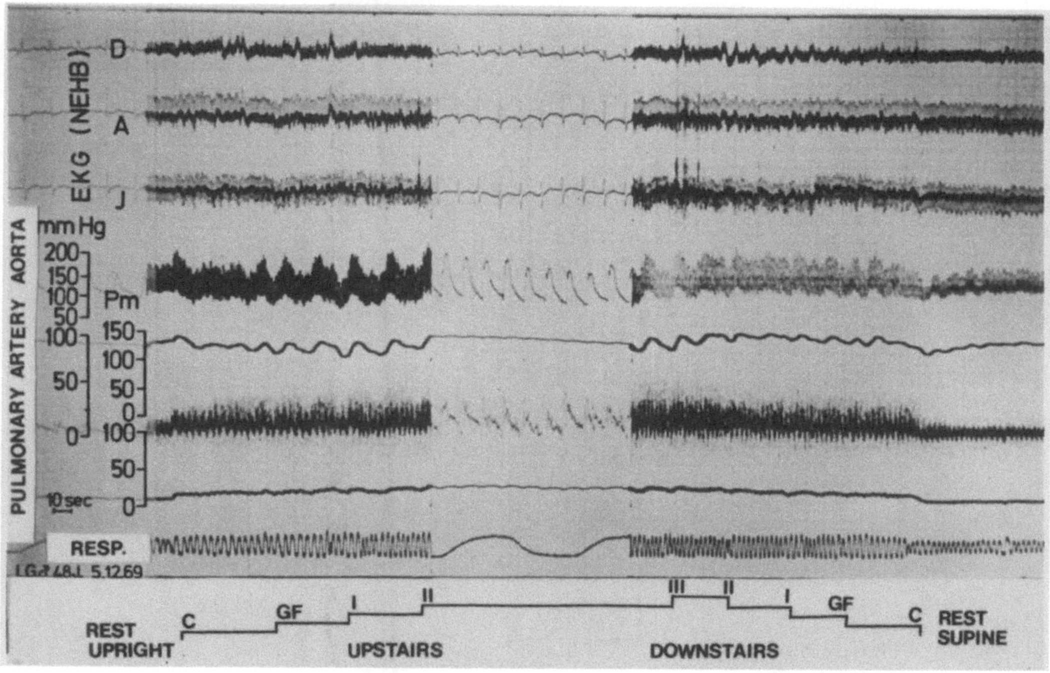

Fig. 2. Multichannel radiotransmission of three leads of the ECG, arterial pressure, pulmonary artery pressure and respiration curve in a 48-year old subject exposed to everyday physical stress

cally rather than medically. ECG telemetry, especially direct tape recording, has the disadvantage of a low signal-to-noise ratio, a reduced lead system, low frequency response, and phase shift [5, 12]. Therefore we performed direct and frequency modulated tape recording of the ECG simultaneously with the 12 standard lead system during exercise stress testing to compare the three methods in the same situation. But the differences observed were only quantitative as far as ST segment depression is concerned and basically inconclusive regarding the diagnosis coronary insufficiency. These findings are in agreement with reports in literature which stated that electromagnetic and radiotelemetered ECG systems allow an accurate clinical evaluation of ischemic ST segment shift [7, 9]. But our results do not confirm the criticism of Hinkle et al. [12], who mentioned the low frequency response and phase shift and stated that the direct recording type of Holter monitoring should not be used for critical ST segment analyses, nor the optimism of Stern and Tzivoni [19], who concluded that 24-h monitoring is more sensitive in detecting silent myocardial ischemia than stress testing. But the fact remains that during daily life situations with fewer periods of submaximal workload, radiotelemetry as well as 24-h storage telemetry of the ECG is less sensitive in detecting myocardial ischemia than exercise testing in the laboratory, with the exception of those rare forms of ischemia not dependent on physical stress such as Prinzmetal's angina or angina to cold. In these situations and

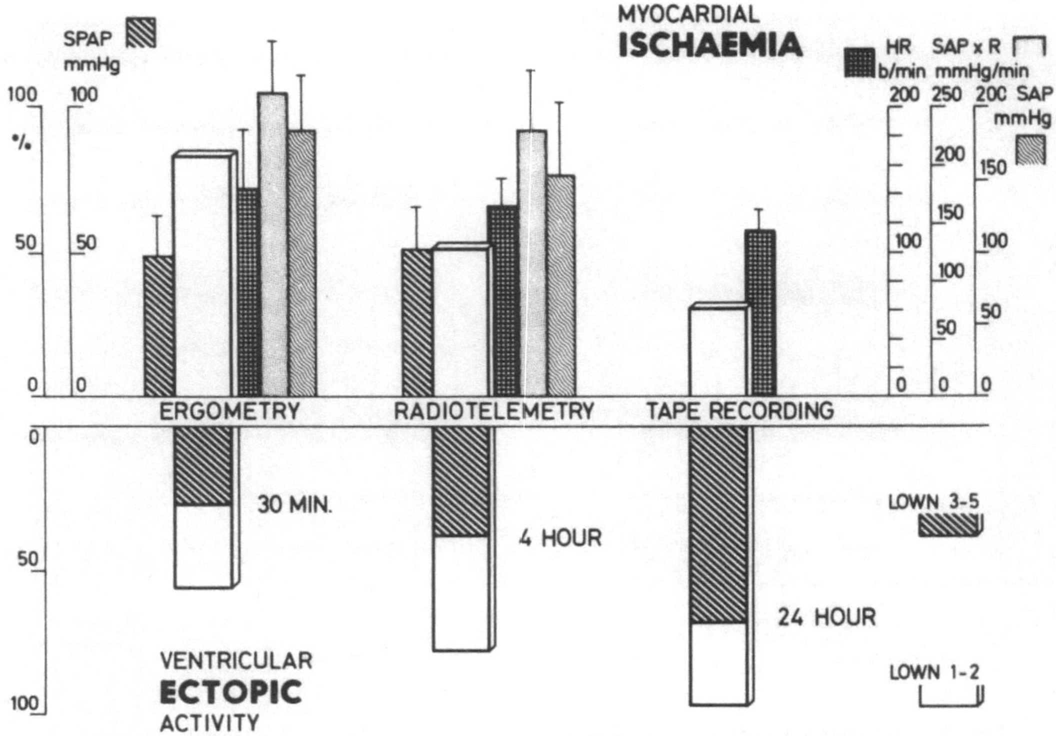

Fig. 3. Sensitivity of ergometry, radiotelemetry and tape recording in detecting coronary heart disease and ventricular ectopic activity in 69 patients with angiographically documented severe coronary lesions

during emotional stress, ECG telemetry may be supplementary in patients with a typical history of angina which is not reproducible and not confirmed by standard exercise testing.

Detection of Ectopic Activity in the Ischemic Myocardium

If one looks at the three methods with respect to their sensitivity in detecting ventricular ectopic activity in coronary heart disease, it seems to be just the other way round. Tape recording over a period of 24 h detects ventricular arrhythmias of grades 1–5 according to Lown's classification [15] in 97% of the cases compared to 73% during a 4-h radiomonitoring and 56% during standard exercise testing with continuous ECG recording over a period of at least 20 min, a 10-min recovery period being included (Fig. 3). Tape recording is not only the most sensitive method in overall sampling of ectopic activity but also in detecting the more serious and thereby prognostically important forms of grades 3–5 in 68% of the cases as compared with 38% by radiotelemetry and 27% by exercise testing. While the so-called significant arrhythmias may occur more episodically tape recording has the greater chance not only in documenting such ventricular ectopic beats but also in detecting couplets, salvos, and R-on-T phenomenon. Long-term prognosis and sudden death are linked to those significant arrhythmias detected during ambulatory monitoring [14, 15]. Therefore, ECG telemetry seems to be superior to the exercise ECG in evaluating the electrically unstable myocardium and thereby prognosis in coronary heart disease.

Radiotelemetry of Direct Blood Pressure Measurements

The Pulmonary Artery and the Arterial System

Another determinant of long-term prognosis in patients with coronary heart disease is given by the left ventricular pump function which is another task of exercise stress testing. But, the general practice of extrapolation from exercise testing in the laboratory on everyday hemodynamic stress in terms of preload, afterload, and rate pressure product has not been checked, however. Therefore the crucial question arises as to the relationship between hemodynamics during stress testing and the cardiovascular response to the hemodynamic stress of everyday situations. This has become one of the main applications of radiotelemetry.

Left Ventricular Pump Failure Preceding Anginal Attack

The well-known work-induced left ventricular pump failure in patients with coronary insufficiency has been demonstrated under daily life situations for the very first time radiotelemetrically. The onset of angina is regularly preceded by a steep increase in pulmonary pressure thereby indicating ischemic left ventricular pump failure which may be prevented by nitrates (Fig. 4). Such studies in even severely ill patients are linked to radiotelemetry, while monitoring the patient at risk on a scope is a must. This prerequisite is not provided by tape recording of direct pressure measurements which have been introduced for use of the arterial system by Beven et al. [6, 13] and widely used ever since by Goldberg et al. [11], Millar-Craig [16], Goldberg and Walsh [18, 10] in analyzing circadian rhythms of arterial blood pressure in normal subjects and in evaluatting medical treatment in patients with arterial hypertension. So at the present state of the art, radiotelemetry transfers invasive methods commonly used in exercise stress testing to daily life situations outside the hospital, these being as accurate as inside the laboratory.

Limitations of Heart Rate Profile in Evaluating Hemodynamic Stress and Cardiac Performance

Everyday hemodynamic stress is very heterogenous as far as dynamic and isometric exercise is concerned. Recommendations concerning the physical training of coronary patients are based on exercise-induced increase of the heart rate mainly, which is measured in the laboratory, monitored in the outpatient radiotelemetrically, recorded on tape or stored by solid state recorders. This policy of focusing on heart rate profiles tends to lead to an underestimation of daily hemodynamic stress in the majority of

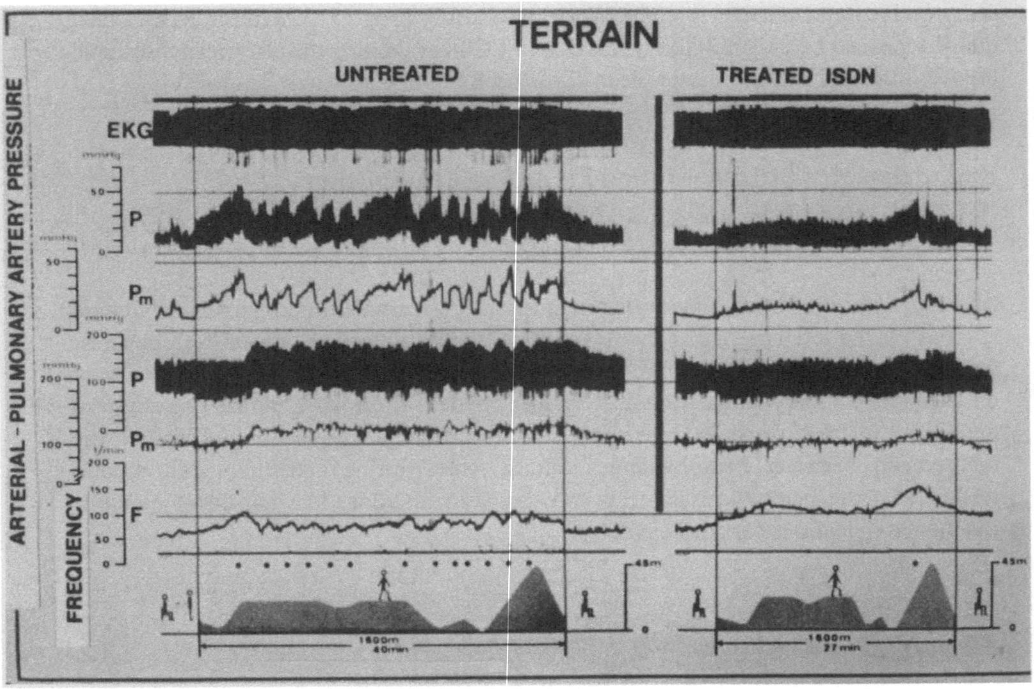

Fig. 4. Recurrent ischemic left ventricular pump failure with abnormal rise in pulmonary artery pressure and concomitant angina (x) in a 47-year old patient during exposure to physical stress before and after sublinqually intake of 10 mg of isosorbid-dinitrate

the situations, especially during isometric work load [20]. This became apparent from a poll in which we asked students, practitioners, and internists to calculate everyday hemodynamic stress as far as heart rate and arterial pressure are concerned (Fig. 5). The exposure of the cardiovascular system to daily life situations is estimated on a level below the radiotelemetric data.

During isometric work load radiotelemetry shows an excessively high diastolic arterial pressure where heart rate is at the lowest. Thus heart rate profile may serve as an indicator of hemodynamic stress during dynamic exercise only and fail completely in guiding the patient when physical training includes dynamic exercise.

Influence of Body Position on Cardiovascular Performance: Underestimation of Working Capacity in the Outpatient by Standard Exercise Testing

There is not only a common underestimation of everyday hemodynamic stress but also an overall underestimation of working capacity by exercise stress testing in patients with impaired cardiovascular function due to coronary heart disease. To assess the prognostic evaluation of working capacity in outpatients by exercise testing we studied 25 patients with coronary insufficiency without myocardial infarction and 17 patients

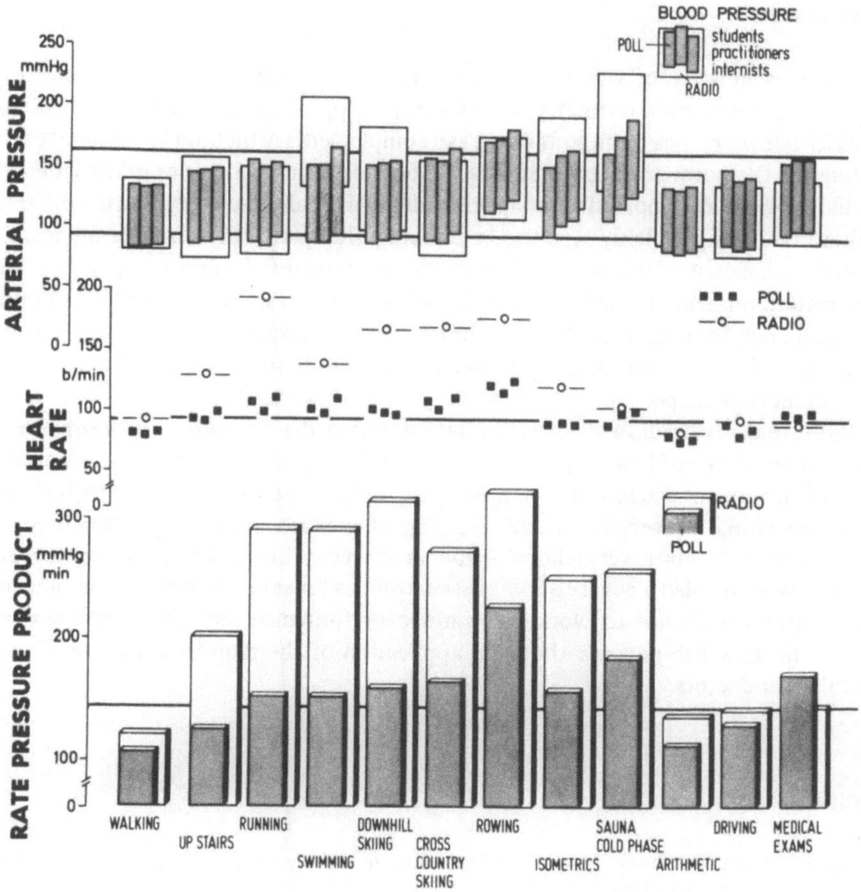

Fig. 5. Hemodynamic stress of everyday activities in terms of arterial pressure, heart rate and double product. Comparison of a general inquiry with radiotelemetric data

with left ventricular aneurysm, with standard bicycle exercise testing in the sitting position and outside the hospital in the terrain [3]. Pulmonary artery pressure and arterial pressure were measured radiotelemetrically and heart rate, rate pressure product, work-load-related diastolic pulmonary artery pressure, and working capacity calculated during ergometry on a bicycle in the supine and sitting positions versus exposure in the terrain. The data in the "ischemic group" as well as in the "aneurysm group" showed working capacity in the terrain to be at its highest while work-load-related diastolic pulmonary artery pressure was at its lowest. As compared to exercise testing in the supine position there is a 13% lower diastolic pulmonary artery pressure with a 113% increase in working tolerance. We conclude from these data that exercising in the supine position is diagnostically highly sensitive in evaluating impairment of left ventricular function, but may fail completely in predicting the working tolerance to exercise as well as everyday hemodynamic stress. Similar results have been reported from graded treadmill exercise [4, 8, 17].

Conclusion

At the present state of the art, telemetry of the cardiovascular system is performed by tape recording, radiotelemetry, transmission by phone, and solid state recordings.

ECG telemetry has to be considered as a complementary method to standard exercise testing. In the coronary patient standard exercise testing is superior in detecting myocardial ischemia as compared with tape recordings and radiotelemetry. On the other hand Holter monitoring is highly sensitive in detecting the electrically unstable myocardium.

Radiotelemetry of direct *blood pressure measurements* facilitates the collection of information on hemodynamic stress and cardiovascular response in everyday situations. As compared to tape recording of direct blood pressure measurements it has the advantage of application in the pulmonary circulation and continuous monitoring of the patient on a scope.

Blood pressure radiotelemetry has demonstrated the limitations of *heart rate profile* as an indicator of hemodynamic stress as well as a predictor of working capacity.

Standard exercise stress testing even with sophisticated methods has its limitations in extrapolating to everyday situations. Type of exercise and body position may differ so extremely during a very short period in everyday life that exercise testing in the laboratory is unable to cover the whole spectrum as far as recommendations concerning the patient's tolerance to work and cardiac performance are concerned. This more prognostic task has become the main application of the radiotransmission of cardiovascular parameters.

References

1 Bachmann K, Thebis J (1967) Die drahtlose Übertragung kontinuierlicher direkter Blutdruckmessungen. Z Kreislaufforsch 56:188

2 Bachmann K, Zerzawy R (1981) Radiotelemetry of direct blood pressure measurements in the arterial and pulmonary system. Biotelemetry and Patient Monitoring (in press)

3 Bachmann K, Zerzawy R (1979) Left ventricular angiography and standard exercise tests in coronary patients as predictors of cardiac performance in daily life. Int symp on haemodynamics and ventricular function during exercise, Berlin, Sept 1979

4 Benge W, Marcus ML (1978) Exercise capacity in patients with scare left ventricular dysfunction. Circulation (Suppl II) 57/58:138

5 Berson AS, Pipberger HV (1966) The low-frequency response of electrocardiographs, a frequent source of recording errors. Am Heart J 71:779

6 Bevan AT, Hunyor, Sleight P, Stott FH (1969) Direct arterial pressure recording in unrestricted man. Clin Sci 36:329

7 Curry RC, Pepine CJ, Conti CR (1979) Ambulatory monitoring to evaluate therapy results in variant angina pectoris. Circulation (Suppl II) 59/60:190

8 Epstein SE, Beiser GD, Stampfer M, Braunwald E (1969) Exercise in patients with heart disease. Effects of body position and type intensity of exercise. Am J Cardiol 23:572

9 Gillian E, Babitt HI, Warabasse JR (1970) Clinical accuracy of ECG ischemic ST-changes recorded by electromagnetic tape (Holter-system) and by radiotelemetry. Circulation (Suppl III) 12/13:111–157

10 Goldberg AD, Walsh T (1979) The analysis of prolonged records of continuous intra-arterial blood pressure – a software approach. ISAM, 3rd Int symp on ambulatory monitoring, Harrow, 1979
11 Goldberg AD, Raftery EB, Cashman PMM, Stott FD (1978) Heart rate, blood pressure correlates in ambulant untreated hypertensive subjects. In: Stott FD, Raftery EB, Sleight P, Gouldin L (eds) ISAM, 2nd Int symp on ambulatory monitoring. Academic Press, London New York San Francisco, p 157
12 Hinkle LE, Meyer J, Stevens M, Carver ST (1967) Tape recordings of the ECG of active men. Limitations and advantages of the Holter-avionics instruments. Circulation 36:752
13 Hunyor SN, Larkin H, Kenny P (1979) The role of ambulatory blood pressure monitoring in assessing efficacy of different anti-hypertensive drug regimes. ISAM 3rd Int symp on ambulatory monitoring, Harrow, 1979
14 Lichtlen PR, Bethge K-P (1980) Beziehungen zwischen malignen ventrikulären Rhythmusstörungen, linksventrikulärer Funktion und plötzlichem Herztod. Verh Dtsch Ges Herz- und Kreislaufforsch 46:27
15 Lown B, Wolf M (1971) Approaches to sudden death from coronary heart disease. Circulation 44:130
16 Millar-Craig MW, Bishop C, Raftery EB (1978) Circadian rhythms of blood pressure in hypertension and modification by drug therapy. ISAM, 2nd Int symp on ambulatory monitoring. Academic Press, London New York San Francisco
17 Niederberger M, Bruce RA, Kusumi F, Whitkanack S (1974) Disparities in ventilatory and circulatory responses to bicycle and treadmill exercise. Br Heart J 36: 377
18 Raftery EB, Millar-Craig MW, Mann St (1981) Long-term ambulatory monitoring of direct blood pressure. Biotelemetry and Patient Monitoring (in press)
19 Stern S, Izivoni D (1974) Early detection of silent ischaemic heart disease by 24-hour electrocardiographic monitoring of active subjects. Br Heart J 36:481
20 Zerzawy R, Bachmann K (1979) Diagnostic and prognostic validity of different types of exercise in coronary heart disease. Int symp on haemodynamics and ventricular function during exercise, Berlin, Sept 1979

Value of Additional Measurements During Exercise Testing: Oxygen Consumption, Blood Pressure, and Cardiac Output

J.M.R. Detry, P. Mairiaux, K. Kandouci, P. Mengeot, J. Melin, and M.F. Rousseau

Introduction

Exercise testing is now routinely used for the diagnosis of coronary artery disease and for the prediction of the severity of the coronary lesions: several chapters of the present book are devoted to these aspects and review the value of exertional electrocardiography (ECG), thallium scintigraphy, and radionuclide angiography.

Besides the ECG data and the isotopic measurements, other parameters can be recorded during exercise testing, namely oxygen consumption, blood pressure, and cardiac output; the value and limitations of these additional measurements will be briefly reviewed in the present chapter.

Oxygen Consumption

The major interest in measuring the oxygen consumption ($\dot{V}_{O_2}$) during an exercise test is to determine the physical working capacity, which is best expressed by the maximal oxygen intake ($\dot{V}_{O_2}$ max) or maximal aerobic capacity [1]. When a subject performs several exercise tests of increasing severity, each separated by a period of rest, there is a linear relationship between oxygen consumption and work load; when the maximal tolerable work load and the exhaustion level are reached there is a trend towards a leveling-off or a plateau in the relationship between the work load and oxygen consumption (Fig. 1). This plateau in oxygen consumption, first described by Hill et al. (1924), is not constantly observed and other signs testify that the subject has reached the $\dot{V}_{O_2}$ max level. These signs are either subjective, such as the exhaustion of a motivated subject, or objective, such as a very elevated heart rate, a high respiratory quotient, and elevated values of blood lactates (Fig. 1). The term $\dot{V}_{O_2}$ max should not be used when these signs are not present and in patients limited by symptoms such as angina pectoris, the term "oxygen consumption limited by symptoms or $\dot{V}_{O_2}$ SL" is preferable [5].

Physiologic Meaning of the Physical Work Capacity

In *healthy subjects,* the $\dot{V}_{O_2}$ max is determined by the physical activity status and it reflects precisely the level of physical fitness. Within the same age group (22–26 years, Table 1), the $\dot{V}_{O_2}$ max goes from 5.6 liters/min in athletes of international class to 4.6 liters/min in athletes of regional class and to 3.1 liters/min in sedentary subjects;

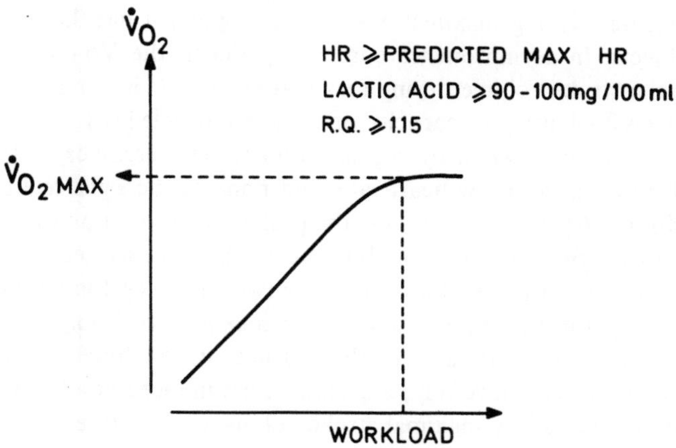

Fig. 1. Relationship between the exercise intensity (*work load*) and the oxygen consumption ($\dot{V}O_2$). When the maximal exercise is reached, the linear relationship often disappears and the $\dot{V}O_2$ does not increase despite a further slight increase in work load: this leveling-off in oxygen consumption corresponds to the maximal aerobic capacity ($\dot{V}O_2$ *max*). Such a plateau in the O_2 consumption is not commonly observed during multistage tests of uninterrupted exercise

these different $\dot{V}O_2$ max values are attended by differences in the stroke volume during maximal exercise. In these subjects, the $\dot{V}O_2$ max is thus an excellent index of the maximal pumping capacity of the left ventricle [15, 16, 30, 32]. The lower $\dot{V}O_2$ max values of older sedentary subjects (Table 1) are mostly due to a decrease in the maximal heart rate with aging and it is not yet known whether or not the stroke volume decreases with increasing age [17]. The same comments apply to women, but in each age or physical activities status group, the $\dot{V}O_2$ max is always lower in women than in men since their stroke volume and maximal arteriovenous difference in oxygen are lower [21].

Coronary patients who are *not limited by angina pectoris* are able to exercise up to their age-predicted maximal heart rate, and elevated values of blood lactates are measured after maximal exercise [25]: in these patients, the $\dot{V}O_2$ max can therefore be

Table 1. Hemodynamic significance of $\dot{V}O_2$ max in healthy men

	Age	$\dot{V}O_2$ max (l/min)	=	HR	x	SV (ml)	x	(A-V) O_2 Difference (ml/100 ml)
Athletes[a]	26	5.6	=	190	x	189	x	15.6
Athletes[b]	25	4.6	=	191	x	149	x	16.1
Sedentary	22	3.1	=	196	x	110	x	14.4
Sedentary	47	2.7	=	182	x	103	x	14.4

[a] Athletes of international class (n = 8).
[b] Athletes of regional class (n = 5). Data calculated from Rowell [29], Ekblom and Hermansen [15], Ekblom et al. [16], Saltin et al. [31], and Hartley et al. [17]

measured during maximal exercise testing and it has the same meaning as in healthy subjects. In asymptomatic coronary patients, the $\dot{V}O_2$ max is also closely correlated to the stroke volume during maximal exercise (Fig. 2) and it is an excellent index of the residual pumping capacity of the left ventricle [12].

In patients *limited by angina pectoris,* the exercise capacity is limited by symptoms which occur at a low heart rate, and none of the signs required for the $\dot{V}O_2$ max are fulfilled [6]. In such patients, the peak O_2 consumption ($\dot{V}O_2$ SL) is an accurate index of their symptom threshold but, due to the great scatter of maximal heart rate, it does not allow a firm conclusion to be drawn regarding the pumping capacity of the heart (Fig. 3). Intuitively, however, a high maximal work load (and $\dot{V}O_2$ SL) attended by a low maximal heart rate (in the absence of beta-blockers) implies an elevated stroke volume while, conversely, angina pectoris induced at a low work load but a high heart rate implies a low maximal stroke volume due to either impaired left ventricular function or excessive sedentariness. In these patients, the physical work capacity is limited by angina pectoris which occurs at a reproducible level of the myocardial oxygen requirements expressed by the pressure-rate product: this index is also a good expression of the severity of the symptoms [25].

Nomographic Assessment of the Physical Working Capacity

The direct measurement of the peak O_2 consumption requires the cooperation of a well-trained technician and the availability of reliable equipment: these two prerequisites are seldom fulfilled and this has led to the development of methods to extrapolate or calculate the physical working capacity. Although useful in population studies and in industrial medicine, all extrapolations of maximal exercise values from submaximal exercise data, as with the nomogram described by Astrand and Ryhming [2], have inherent limitations which have been discussed elsewhere [1, 31].

The calculation of the physical work capacity from the maximal work load has been recommended by Bruce and is based on a close relationship existing between the maximal work load and the peak oxygen intake [3]; this approach requires the use of a fully standardized exercise protocol and, ideally, normal values should be available so that the results can be expressed with reference to the normal expected values for subjects of the same age and sex. Since the treadmill remains unpopular in Europe, we have collected data in normal subjects submitted to a standardized bicycle exercise test starting at 20 W during 1 min with subsequent increments of 20 W every minute; this slope has been chosen rather than a lower one (10 W/min) since it permits testing with a reasonable time, and, accordingly, to exactly the same protocol, severely limited patients as well as healthy subjects. With this protocol, there is, as expected, a linear relationship between the work load and the O_2 consumption (Fig. 4); as previously observed, at every exercise intensity, the O_2 consumption is slightly lower in women than in men [1, 3]. From the data presented in Fig. 4, it is possible to calculate, in a given subject, the $\dot{V}O_2$ max or the $\dot{V}O_2$ SL from the maximal work load: this approach has been tested in 100 patients and the calculated peak $\dot{V}O_2$ slightly underestimates the directly measured peak $\dot{V}O_2$ (- 60 ml/min; - 3%; N.S.). The normal values of $\dot{V}O_2$ max and maximal work load are presented in Fig. 5 which shows the expected decrease in $\dot{V}O_2$ max with age; the $\dot{V}O_2$ max is always higher in men than in women. From

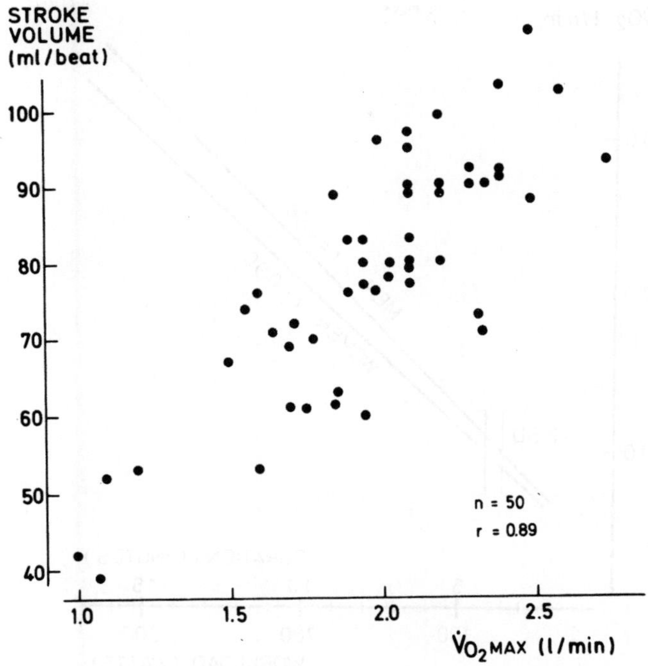

Fig. 2. Relationship between the maximal oxygen intake ($\dot{V}O_2$ *max*) and the stroke volume during maximal exercise in 50 coronary patients not limited by exertional angina pectoris

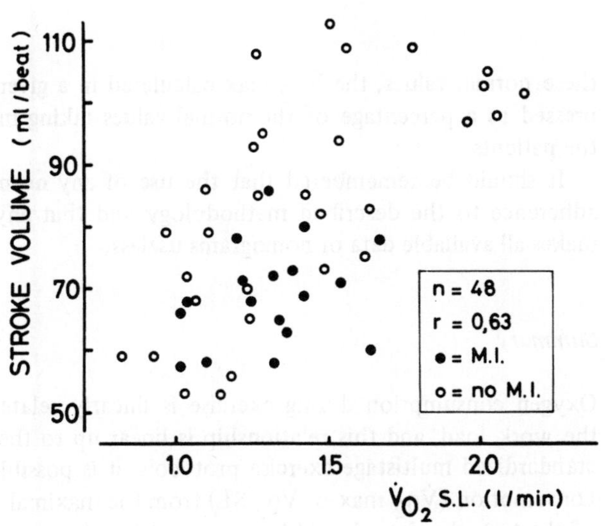

Fig. 3. Relationship between the symptom-limited peak oxygen consumption ($\dot{V}O_2 SL$) and the stroke volume during maximal exercise in 48 coronary patients limited by exertional angina pectoris. *MI*, myocardial infarction

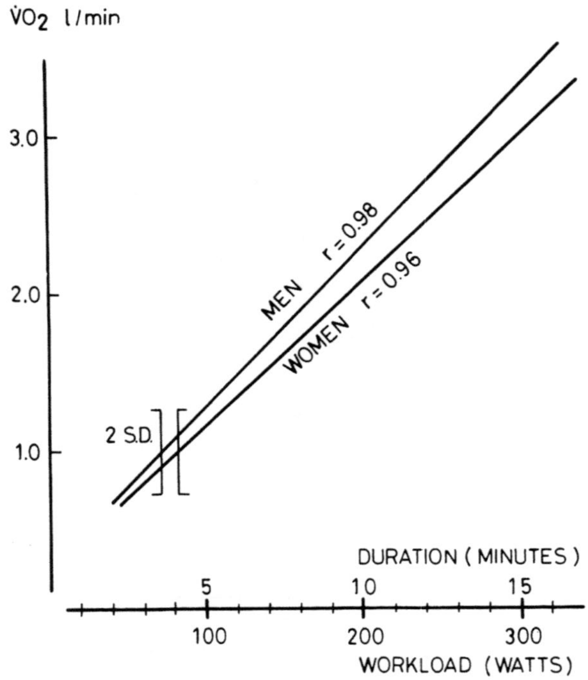

Fig. 4. Oxygen consumption during a multistage bicycle exercise test with an inititial work load of 20 W for 1 min and subsequent increments of 20 W every minute: data calculated from 586 measurements in 80 men and 587 measurements in 80 women. From these relationships, it is easy to calculate the $\dot{V}_{O_2}$ *max* or the $\dot{V}_{O_2}$ *SL* from the maximal work load

these normal values, the $\dot{V}_{O_2}$ max calculated in a given patient or subject can be expressed as a percentage of the normal values taking into account the age and sex of the patients.

It should be remembered that the use of any normalized protocol requires strict adherence to the described methodology and that any modification of the protocol makes all available data or nomograms useless.

Summary

Oxygen consumption during exercise is linearly related to the exercise intensity or the work load, and this relationship is linear up to the maximal exercise level. Using standardized multistage exercise protocols, it is possible to calculate the peak oxygen consumption ($\dot{V}_{O_2}$ max or $\dot{V}_{O_2}$ SL) from the maximal work load or the total duration of the test; the data should be expressed in reference to data collected in normal subjects (percentage of normal expected values or functional aerobic impairment). This nomographic approach provides an accurate measurement of the physical work capacity and is to be recommended in clinical practice. It should be mentioned here that many

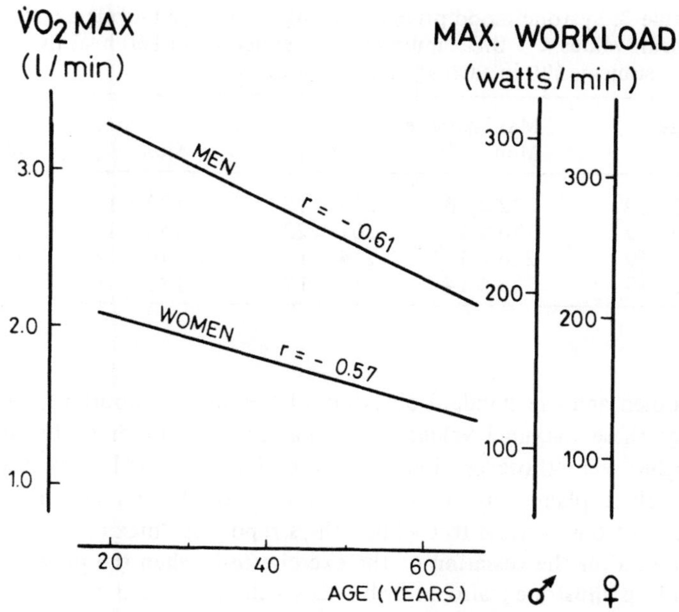

Fig. 5. Normal values of maximal oxygen consumption (*left*) and maximal work load (*right*) in healthy men (*n*, 80) and women (*n*, 80); age from 20–60. Data collected during a multistage bicycle exercise test with an initial work load of 20 W for 1 min and subsequent increments of 20 W every minute

patients prefer to exercise without the masks or mouthpieces required for the direct measurement and that this facilitates dialogue with the patient during the test itself.

Where clinical research is concerned, it is often preferable to measure directly the oxygen consumption and the carbon dioxide excretion (open or closed circuits); these measurements are mandatory when the Fick principle is used to determined the cardiac output at rest or during exercise.

Blood Pressure

Most authors recommend the measurement of blood pressure (cuff method) at rest before the test and then during the test itself at regular intervals including at the maximal exercise level. During exercise, it is often difficult to measure reliably diastolic pressure and the value of the diastolic pressure will not be discussed here.

Maximal Systolic Blood Pressure

Table 2 presents the systolic blood pressure measured at the maximal exercise level in 160 normal subjects subdivided according to age and sex into eight groups of 20 subjects each; all subjects were normotensive at rest (BP < 145/85 mm Hg). The values obtained at the maximal exercise level are extremely high, 10–20 mm Hg lower in

Table 2. Systolic blood pressure during multistage bicycle exercise testing (mean values ± 1 S.D.; mmHg); data collected in 160 healthy normotensive subjects (20 in each age and sex group)

Age	Maximal exercise		Early recovery	
	Men	Women	Men	Women
20–29	232 ± 16	213 ± 17	177 ± 15	161 ± 15
30–39	236 ± 19	201 ± 22	158 ± 17	167 ± 15
40–49	226 ± 15	214 ± 17	176 ± 18	170 ± 21
50–59	225 ± 14	212 ± 17	186 ± 16	178 ± 25

women and the standard deviation of the data is important, ranging from 15–20 mm Hg; these maximal values are similar to those observed by Mallion et al. [22] but higher than those previously reported by others [4]. This discrepancy seems to be largely explained by the fact that our measurements have been made during the last 15 s of the exercise test while others report as "maximal" the systolic pressure measured after the cessation of the exercise test, when the pressure is quickly decreasing. This is illustrated also in Table 2 which shows that the systolic pressure measured 1 min after the end of the exercise test is much lower than the maximal systolic pressure. Our data suggest that age does not significantly influence the maximal systolic pressure which is in agreement with other reports [20]. It is important to note, however, that although the maximal systolic blood pressure seems unaffected by aging, the simultaneous maximal heart rate goes down from 195–175 in men and from 194–174 in women.

The cuff method is known to overestimate systolic blood pressure during exercise. In a different group of 12 young healthy subjects we have measured systolic brachial pressure both invasively and noninvasively with the cuff method: the "invasive" maximal systolic pressure was always 15–20 mm Hg lower than the pressure measured by the cuff method [17].

Interpretation of the Pressure Response to Exercise

During a multistage test, the systolic blood pressure response is closely related to the heart rate (Fig. 6); this relationship is slightly different in the women who have a less marked increase in blood pressure during exercise. This observation indicates that the pressure response to exercise cannot be analyzed without taking into account the concomitant heart rate: only the values falling outside the ± 2 standard deviation limit should be considered as abnormal.

In subjects who are normotensive at rest, it is exceptional to measure a blood pressure falling above the normal limits and the meaning of these "abnormalities" is unclear. In hypertensive patients, the maximal systolic blood pressure tends to be higher than in normals, but the changes in pressure from the resting values are slightly less [4]. Although these differences are statistically significant, the values measured in normals widely overlap those measured in hypertensive patients and an individual measurement is therefore exceedingly difficult to interpret.

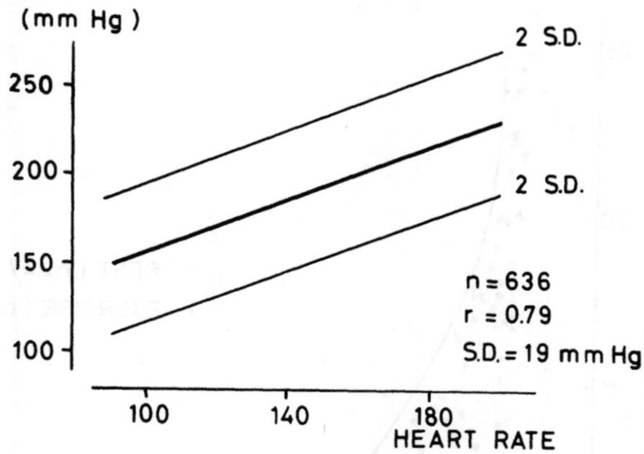

Fig. 6. Systolic blood pressure during a multistage bicycle exercise test (20 W/min) in 80 healthy men; note the close relationship with the heart rate

A poor pressure response to exercise or a fall in blood pressure during exercise is sometimes observed and it has been considered as an indication to interrupt the exercise test [19]. Such a poor pressure response to exercise is infrequent: of the coronary patients reported by Irving at al. [20] only 16% demonstrated such a response and this would probably have been much less if patients limited by angina pectoris at low exercise level had been excluded from this study. This type of pressure response simply reflects a poor left ventricular function and these patients most often have other clinical signs of left ventricular dysfunction such as a cardiomegaly and a history of previous severe myocardial infarction and/or heart failure. The prognostic value of this finding has been advocated by Irving et al. [20], who reported that the maximal blood pressure below 140 mm Hg was a specific (89%) but poorly sensitive (39%) predictor of subsequent sudden cardiac death; the predictive value (percentage of patients with this finding and subsequently dying) is only 21%. A low pressure response to exercise does not seem to provide important additional information in a significant subset of patients. In the absence of other clinical signs or symptoms, we doubt that it is a clear-cut indication for interrupting an exercise test.

Summary

To summarize, it is useful to measure systolic blood pressure during an exercise test but the information provided by this measurement is limited and the diastolic readings are most often unreliable. When the blood pressure response to exercise is a major issue in an individual, the only way to solve the problem is to measure it invasively and to calculate the systemic resistance by measuring simultaneously the cardiac output; the recorded data will then be compared to normal reference values as presented in Fig. 7.

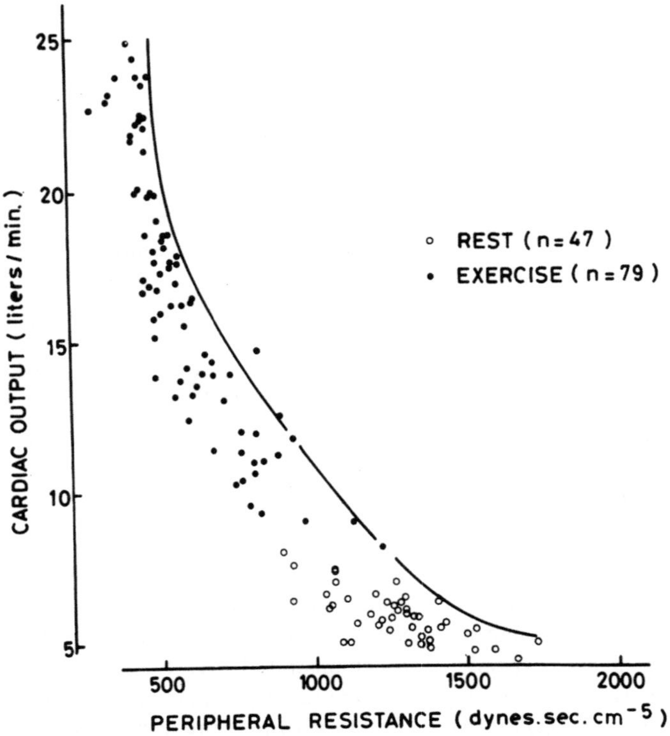

Fig. 7. Peripheral resistance at rest and during exercise (data collected in 21 nomal young subjects); the line of normal limits has been drawn visually and not calculated (from Detry el al. [8, 11])

Cardiac Output

Methodology

Cardiac output can be measured either with the Fick method or with a dye-dilution technique. Both methods are equally effective, but the Fick principle is interesting because it requires the placing of a catheter in the mean pulmonary artery and allows easy measurements of the pulmonary and capillary wedge pressures. The catheter should be introduced in the least traumatic way, i.e., percutaneously, so that no vessel repairs and skin sutures are needed. We use a Swan-Ganz catheter, which is placed through a small Teflon tube (Desilet), and a small Teflon catheter for brachial artery. These manipulations are easy and fast but they require good training.

The quality of the measurements requires a relative hemodynamic steady state so that each exercise level should be maintained 4–5 min before increasing the work load to a higher exercise level. After collection of the baseline resting data with the patients in an upright position, our patients perform at a minimum of two exercise levels, each for 5 min: one low exercise level (± 50% of the physical work capacity) and one maximal exercise level. The work loads corresponding to these exercise levels are chosen according to the results of a prior test of maximal exercise. The risks in these studies are very low and among hundreds of such procedures we had no major complications; this does not mean, however, that these hemodynamic studies are pleasant and totally painless for the patients.

Interpretation of the Data Collected in Coronary Patients

During *submaximal exercise,* requiring approximately 60% of the physical capacity of the patients, cardiac output is most often normal in coronary patients; among 130 patients (Fig. 8), cardiac output fell within the normal expected values in 80% of the cases. These normal limits have been calculated from 133 measurements made in 15 normal young subjects who have been repeatedly catheterized [8, 11]. An abnormal cardiac output during submaximal exercise was observed in only 26 patients; 21 of whom (80%) had had previous myocardial infarction. These patients with an abnormal cardiac output response tend to have a lower resting ejection fraction, more extensive coronary artery disease, and more damaged left ventricles. From a normal cardiac output during submaximal exercise, it is, however, impossible to predict accurately the extent of the coronary lesions, or the state of the resting left ventricular function.

During *maximal exercise,* limited by angina pectoris or by exhaustion, cardiac output is abnormal in approximately 50% of the patients (53 of 104, Fig. 9); such an

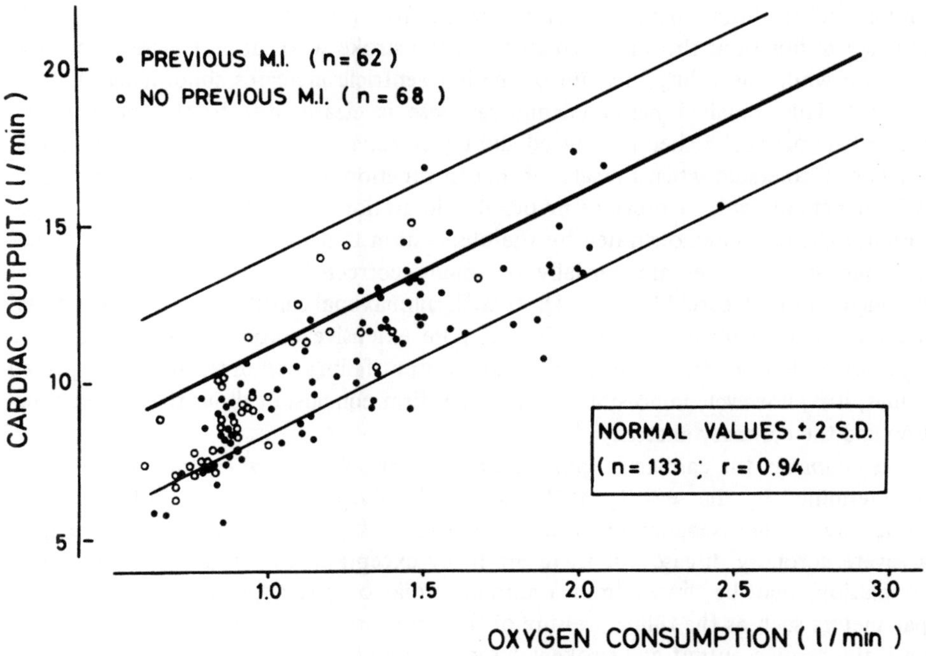

Fig. 8. Cardiac output during submaximal exercise in 130 coronary patients. *MI,* myocardial infarction

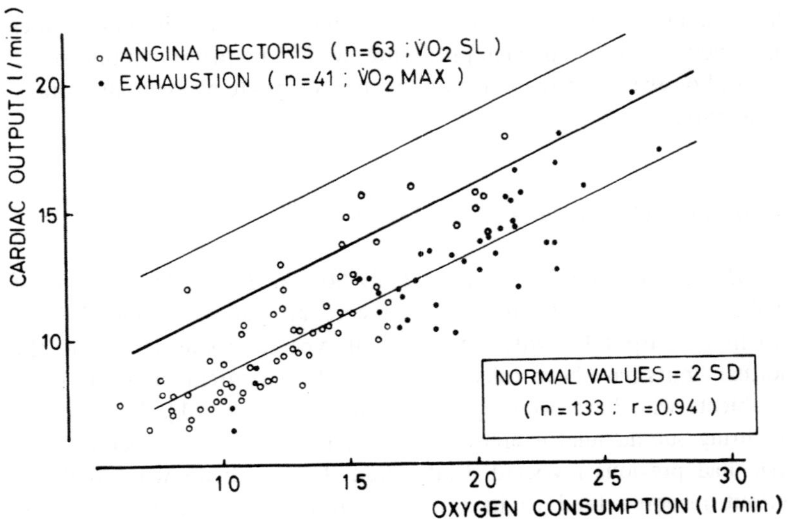

Fig. 9. Cardiac output during maximal exercise in 104 coronary patients

abnormal response is as frequent in patients limited by angina pectoris (33/63; 52%) as it is in patients limited by exhaustion (20/41; 49%). Interestingly, but not indicated in Fig. 9, the majority of the patients with an abnormally low maximal cardiac output have a previous myocardial infarction (38 of 53, 72%). This abnormal behavior of the cardiac output during maximal exercise results from a transient depression of the left ventricular function; the stroke volume and the stroke work do not increase or even decrease while the filling pressure of the left ventricle increases abnormally [12, 23, 24, 26]. This impaired hemodynamic response is clearly due to the more or less marked myocardial ischemia induced during maximal exercise testing. This ischemia is less well tolerated when the left ventricular function is already impaired at rest than it is in patients with a previous myocardial infarction [12]. The causal role of myocardial ischemia is demonstrated by the observation that in coronary patients, hemodynamic abnormalities are partially or totally corrected by the administration of sublingual nitroglycerin [10, 12, 24]. As with submaximal cardiac output, an abnormal maximal cardiac output is indicative of more extensive coronary lesions and more myocardial damage; from a maximal cardiac output falling within the normal expected values, it is, however, impossible to draw any firm conclusion about the cardiac function and the coronary anatomy.

In *summary*, the cardiac output response during submaximal and maximal exercise is determined by the severity of the disease already present at rest and by the additional myocardial ischemia induced by the stress test; an abnormal response suggests a severe coronary disease but there are many exceptions to this general rule and no conclusions may be drawn from a normal cardiac output response. Of course, other parameters such as the filling pressure of the left ventricle should be analyzed together with the cardiac output and stroke volume response to exercise. These parameters add some useful information but in a given patient, the clinical usefulness of hemodynamic measurements during exercise appears to be limited.

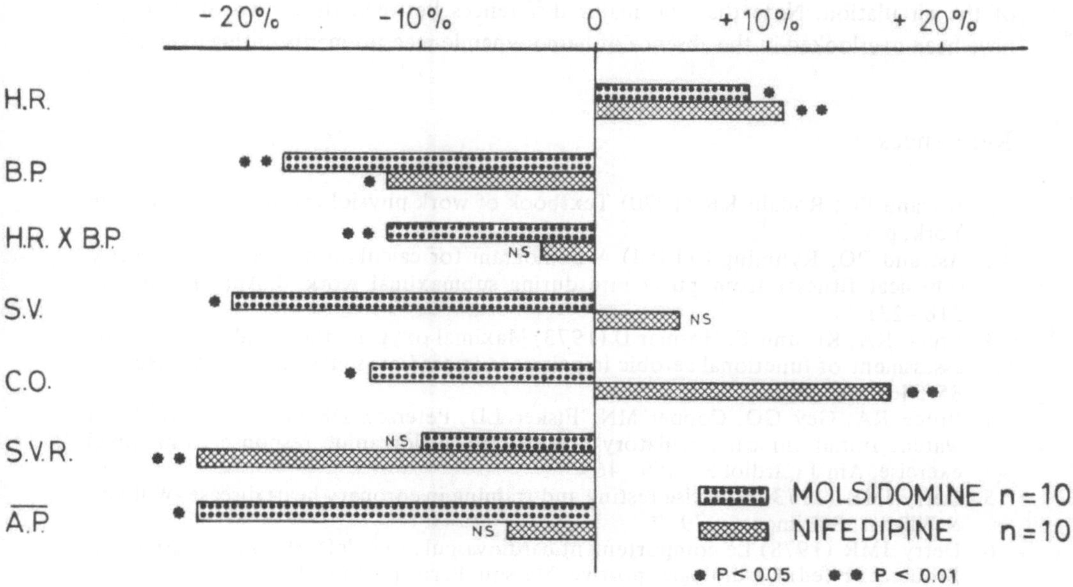

Fig. 10. Hemodynamic modifications observed in coronary patients during submaximal exercise performed 1 h after administration of Molsidomine (2 mg i.v.) or nifedipine (20 mg per os); from Detry et al. [13, 14]. *HR*, heart rate; *BP*, blood pressure; *SV*, stroke volume; *CO*, cardiac output; *SVR*, systems vascular resistances; *AP*, mean pulmonary arterial pressure

Interest in Clinical Research

Because of the difficulties in interpreting the hemodynamic data collected during exercise in a given patient, we think that such studies have a limited clinical value; the place of these invasive measurements during exercise is, however, unique in clinical research when a patient is investigated before and after a therapeutic intervention. That intervention can be medical or surgical and the delay between the measurements may vary from 1 h to several months [7, 9, 10, 11, 13, 14, 26, 27, 28, 29, 33].

Figure 10 illustrates the interesting aspects of hemodynamic measurements during exercise in the assessment of the mechanisms of action of two drugs recently proposed for the treatment of angina pectoris: Molsidomine, which is a nitrate-like drug, and nifedipine, which is a calcium antagonist [13, 14]. Both drugs cause a decrease in blood pressure and an increase in heart rate and at first glance they might look similar. These drugs have, however, opposite effects on the cardiac output. Molsidomine induces a significant decrease in cardiac output, stroke volume, and mean pulmonary arterial pressure: these effects suggest a predominant action on the venous capacitance with a decreased venous return. The lower blood pressure after Molsidomine appears to result mostly from a decreased cardiac output with no change in peripheral resistance. Nifedipine causes an important increase in cardiac output that probably results from the major decrease in the systemic vascular resistance which explains the lower blood pressure; thus, this calcium antagonist acts mainly as a dilator of the arterial side of the circulation. Note that the major differences between these two drugs might have been overlooked in the absence of hemodynamic measurements during exercise.

References

1 Astrand PO, Rodahl KR (1970) Textbook of work physiology. McGrae-Hill, New York, p 669

2 Astrand PO, Ryhming I (1954) A nomogram for calculation of aerobic capacity (physical fitness) from pulse rate during submaximal work. J Appl Physiol 7: 218–221

3 Bruce RA, Kusumi F, Hosmer D (1973) Maximal oxygen intake and nomographic assessment of functional aerobic impairment in cardiovascular disease. Am Heart J 85:546–562

4 Bruce RA, Gey GO, Cooper MN, Fisher LD, Peterson DR (1974) Seattle heart watch: Initial clinical circulatory and electrocardiographic response to maximal exercise. Am J Cardiol 33:459–469

5 Detry JMR (1973) Exercise testing and training in coronary heart disease. Williams & Wilkins, Baltimore, p 79

6 Detry JMR (1978) Le comportement cardiovasculaire à l'effort du coronarien. In: Broustet JP (ed) Cardiologie sportive. Masson, Paris, pp 153–164

7 Detry JMR, Rousseau M, Vandenbroucke G, Kusumi F, Brasseur LA, Bruce RA (1971) Increased arterio-venous oxygen difference after physical training in coronary heart disease. Circulation 44:109–118

8 Detry JMR, Gerin M, Charlier A, Brasseur LA (1972) Hemodynamic aspects of prolonged "intermittent" exercise. Int Z Angew Physiol 30:171–185

9 Detry JMR, Rousseau MF, Brasseur LA (1975) Early hemodynamic adaptations to physical training in patients with healed myocardial infarction. Eur J Cardiol 2:307–313

10 Detry JMR, Rousseau MF, Filleul P, Brasseur LA (1975) Effects of nitroglycerin on the hemodynamic response to maximal exercise in coronary patients limited by exertional angina pectoris (Abstract). Eur J Clin Invest (Suppl 1) 7: Vol 5:7

11 Detry JMR, Rousseau MF, Filleul P, Frans A, Clerbaux Th, Brasseur LA (1976) Hemodynamic effects of lidoflazine during graded levels of bicycle exercise in normal subjects. Eur J Cardiol 4:165–174

12 Detry JMR, Mengeot P, Brasseur LA, Cosyns J, Rousseau MF (1978) Ventricular function in coronary heart disease. Adv Cardiol 24:37–46

13 Detry JMR, Melin J, Brasseur LA, Cosyns J, Rousseau MF (1981) Hemodynamic effects of Molsidomine at rest, during submaximal and maximal exercise in coronary patients limited by exertional angina pectoris. Am J Cardiol 47:109

14 Detry JMR, Melin J, Brasseur LA, Cosyns J, Rousseau MF (to be published) Hemodynamic effects of nifedipine at rest, during submaximal and maximal exercise in coronary patients limited by exertional angina pectoris

15 Ekblom B, Hermansen L (1968) Cardiac output in athletes. J Appl Physiol 25: 619–625

16 Ekblom B, Astrand PO, Saltin B, Stenberg J, Wallström B (1968) Effects of training on the circulatory response to exercise. J Appl Physiol 24:518–528

17 Hartley LH, Grimby G, Kiblom A, Nilsson NJ, Astrand I, Bjure J, Ekblom B, Saltin B (1969) Physical training in sedentary middle-aged and older men. III. Cardiac output and gas exchange at submaximal and maximal exercise. Scand J Clin Lab Invest 24:335–344

18 Hill A, Long C, Lupton H (1924) Muscular exercise, lactic acid and the supply and ultilization of oxygen. Proc Roy Soc London 96:438–475

19 Irving JB, Bruce RA (1977) Exertional hypotension and postexertional ventricular fibrillation in stress testing. Am J Cardiol 39:849–851

20 Irving JB, Bruce RA, DeRouen TA (1977) Variations in and significance of systolic pressure during maximal exercise (treadmill) testing. Relation to severity of coronary artery disease and cardiac mortality. Am J Cardiol 39:841–848
21 Kiblom A, Astrand I (1971) Physical training with submaximal intensities in women. II. Effect on cardiac output. Scand J Clin Lab Invest 28:163–175
22 Mallion JM, Debru JL, Mikler F, Avezou F, Cau G, Muller JM (1974) Mesure du profil tensionnel d'effort normal. Applications pratiques chez l'hypertendu. Nouv Presse Med 3:2003–2006
23 McCans JL, Parker JO (1973) Left ventricular pressure volume relationship during myocardial ischemia in man. Circulation 48:775–785
24 Parker JO, West RO, Di Giorgi S (1967) The hemodynamic response to exercise in patients with healed myocardial infarction without angina. With observations on the effects of nitroglycerin. Circulation 36:734–751
25 Robinson BF (1967) Relation of heart rate and systolic blood pressure to the onset of the pain in angina pectoris. Circulation 35:1073–1083
26 Rousseau M, Brasseur LA, Detry JMR (1973) Hemodynamic determinants of maximal oxygen intake in patients with healed myocardial infarction; influence of physical training. Circulation 48:943–949
27 Rousseau MF, Brasseur LA, Detry JMR (1973) Haemodynamic and electrocardiographic effects of practolol during upright exercise in coronary heart disease. Cardiovascular Res 7:306–312
28 Rousseau MF, Brasseur LA, Detry JMR (1973) Effects of a new oral antiarrhythmic drug (Aprindine) on the hemodynamic response to upright exercise. Acta Cardiol (Brux) 28:456–462
29 Rousseau MF, Degre S, Messin R, Brasseur LA, Denolin H, Detry JMR (1974) Hemodynamic effects of early physical training after acute myocardial infarction; comparison with a control untrained group. Eur J Cardiol 2:39–45
30 Rowell LB (1962) Factors affecting the prediction of the maximal oxygen intake from measurements made during submaximal work with observations related to factors which may limit maximal oxygen intake. Ph D thesis, University of Minnesota, p 275
31 Rowell LB, Taylor HL, Wang Y (1964) Limitations to prediction of maximal oxygen intake. J Appl Physiol 19:919–927
32 Saltin B, Blomquist GM, Mitchell JH, Johnson RL, Wildenthal K, Chapman CB (1968) Response to exercise after bedrest and after training. Circulation (Suppl 7) 38:78
33 Serruys PW, Rousseau MF, Cosyns J, Ponlot R, Brasseur LA, Detry JMR (1978) Hemodynamics during maximal exercise after coronary bypass surgery. Br Heart J 40:1205–1215

Indications for Electrocardiographic Exercise Testing in the Detection of Ischemic Myocardium

M.H. Frick

Introduction

When done properly, i.e. obeying established contraindications and indications for stopping the test, exercise testing is a remarkable safe procedure. In extensive multicenter experience mortality has ranged from 0.005% to 0.01% and morbidity in terms of arrhythmias and prolonged chest pain necessitating hospitalization, from 0.04%–0.08% [7, 19]. The author's personal experience over the last 10 years covers some 500 tests with two cases of transient pathologic Q-waves (0.04%). Despite this, safety indications for exercise testing in the detection of ischemic myocardium should be clearly defined. This is essential both in terms of cost/benefit and to avoid vague information. Economical aspects are not crucial in the cost/benefit analysis, but the manpower involved is considerable since maximal testing should not be performed without an attending physician. Equivocal information from indiscriminant use of exercise testing is distressing for the physician and test subjects alike.

The indications for exercise testing can be divided into two categories: (1) the detection of ischemic heart disease and (2) quantitation of manifest ischemic heart disease in terms of exercise tolerance as shown in the following list:

I. The detection of ischemic heart disease

1. Asymptomatic individuals
   Pilots
   "Coronary-prone" subjects
   Population samples in epidemiology
   Middle-aged individuals before physical training programs
   Insurance problems
2. Subjects with chest pain
   Heberdeen's angina pectoris
   Variant angina pectoris
   "Noncoronary" pain
3. Demonstration of exercise-related ventricular arrhythmias
   Triggering of diagnostic ventricular ectopics in the presence of intraventricular conduction disturbance

II. Determination of exercise tolerance

1. Evaluation of postinfarction patients
2. Before and after physical training programs
3. Follow-up of medical and surgical therapy
4. Assessment of capacity for work

The Detection of Ischemic Heart Disease

Testing of Asymptomatic Individuals

This poses two problems. The first is related to the validity of the test result, the second is an ethical dilemma. During recent years it has become evident that both the sensitivity and specificity of the test are dependent not only on the form and degree of electrocardiographic changes but also on the conditional probability of the test (Bayes' theorem). This theorem states that the test result cannot be adequately interpreted without reference to the prevalence of the disease in the population under study. This pretest likelihood of having the disease is low in an asymptomatic population. The statistical thesis of Bayes has been applied to some exercise test data with clear establishment of the fact that the predictive accuracy is related to the pretest likelihood of coronary artery disease [6, 18]. This relationship cannot be circumvented by increasing the criterion for the degree of accepted ST segment depression from 1 mm to, for example, 3 mm since this leads to a decreased sensitivity of the test [8]. The ethical problem arises from the impact of a positive result on the test subject. Even if the result is a "true positive" one the preventive and therapeutic implications are hazy. There is no firm evidence that any preventive, medical, or surgical measures would improve the posttest prognosis. On the contrary, the knowledge of having a coronary heart disease can have disastrous psychological effects on the individual concerned.

In light of the problems briefly outlined above, testing of asymptomatic individuals should be restricted to certain groups. One of these consists of subjects responsible for other people's safety, such as airline pilots. Periodic exercise testing is recommended and in general use [12]. Subjects with multiple risk factors including bad family history ("coronary-prone" individuals) can be subjected to exercise testing especially upon request. It is presumably useful to test middle-aged individuals before they embark on physical conditioning programs. One group of subjects whose testing is justified are "asymptomatic" individuals who have problems related to getting insurance.

In order to analyze the prevalence of ischemic heart disease in a population sample, exercise testing can be used with clear understanding of the problems outlined in connection with testing of asymptomatic individuals. Maximal stressing should be applied since, as discussed previously [10], the use of submaximal standard loads may lead to the false impression of physically fit individuals having a low prevalence of coronary heart disease.

Testing of Subjects with Chest Pain

This subgroup is the largest and includes pain syndromes suggestive of ischemic heart disease and clearly "noncoronary" pain. In the latter variety exercise testing is often curative. Demonstration of myocardial ischemia, even in classical Heberdeen's angina, is desirable if the results of therapeutic interventions are to be related to attenuation of ischemia. This practice concerns both medical and surgical treatments. Exercise testing is also a part of the evaluation of patients with suspected or proven coronary artery spasm. Recently a group of patients was described who had coronary artery spasms and exercise-induced ST segment shifts when tested early in the morning but not in the afternoon [26], demonstrating the advantage of testing according to medical history.

Demonstration of Exercise-Induced Arrhythmias

This is one of the testing indications. This includes triggering of the arrhythmias per se and creation of diagnostic ventricular ectopics in cases where ischemic heart disease is masked by the presence of aberrant ventricular conduction [1]. There has been some disagreement over the clinical significance of exercise-induced ventricular arrhythmias or the disappearance of ectopics during exercise [4, 5, 13, 14, 15, 25]. The consensus regarding the significance of exercise-related ventricular ectopics was recently summarized as follows: (1) in apparently healthy individuals the presence of ventricular ectopics without associated ST segment depression is of little or no prognostic significance, and (2) subjects with both significant ST segment shift and ventricular arrhythmias are likely to have a severe coronary artery disease [7]. It thus seems probable that the use of exercise is useful both in the clarification of patients' symptoms related to ventricular arrhythmias and to afford additional evidence for the severity of coronary heart disease. Opinions differ on the superiority of 24-h Holter monitoring as compared to exercise testing [17, 20]. If exercise is triggering arrhythmias in a given individual the difference in the prevalence between long-term monitoring and exercise test is evidently related to the number of periods of physical effort during the monitoring. Data on the repeatability of effort-induced ectopics are so far scanty. Nevertheless, repetitive exercise testing can be used in monitoring of antiarrhythmic therapy.

Quantitation of Exercise Tolerance in Manifest Ischemic Heart Disease

The Pros and Cons of Testing Patients with Acute Myocardial Infarction at Discharge

These have been evaluated by a number of studies [2, 9, 22, 23]. The consensus is that low-level stress testing is feasible and safe provided certain precautions are taken. The patients must be free of cardiac failure, uncontrolled ventricular arrhythmias, and atrioventricular conduction disturbances. The effect of a number of drugs such as digitalis, antihypertensives, diuretics, and beta-adrenergic blocking compounds should be taken into account in the interpretation of test results. When carried out and interpreted properly the test seems to give useful information on the subsequent prognosis of the patient [24]. This may help in intensifying therapy for the patients at high risk but so far controlled studies are lacking.

Assessment of Exercise Tolerance

The aim is to determine the patient's ability to cope with the demands of his job, to evaluate the effect of drug therapy in terms of both its validity and side effects, and to assess the effect of surgical interventions. The energy expenditure of different jobs in terms of ergometric/treadmill loads or oxygen consumption is well known and form the basis for the evaluation of patients' ability or disability in everyday life. It has been suggested that the validity of treatment with beta-adrenergic blocking drugs should be evaluated by peak exercise heart rates [16], but in routine clinical practice exercise testing is not mandatory in the follow-up of medical therapy. On the other hand, when coronary bypass surgery is considered exercise stress data are extremely useful when making decisions. In the first place, they demonstrate whether angiographically visualized coronary artery obstructions have myocardial consequences. Secondly, the preoperative stress data are very useful in the long-term follow-up of the operated patient. Innumerable coronary bypass studies have been made using only functional classification, which is prone to several inaccuracies.

Determination of exercise tolerance is an inherent procedure in physical training programs for patients with manifest ischemic heart disease [3, 11, 21].

This brief survey of the indications for exercise testing in the detection of ischemic myocardium includes only electrocardiographic monitoring. Exercise can also be applied to the detection of myocardial ischemia by other monitoring systems, e.g., coronary sinus lactate sampling, isotope scanning, and cineangiography.

References

1 Anttonen V-M, Oka M, Holopainen T (1959) Diagnostic significance of ventricular premature beats in acute myocardial infarction. Ann Med Intern Fenn (Suppl 29) 48:1–30
2 Atterhög J-H, Ekelund L-G, Kaijser L (1971) Electrocardiographic abnormalities during exercise 3 weeks to 18 months after anterior myocardial infarction. Br Heart J 33:871–877
3 Clausen JP, Larsen OA, Trap-Jensen J (1969) Physical training in the management of coronary artery disease. Circulation 40:143–154
4 Cohn K (1976) Interpretation and limitations in stress testing. Adv Cardiol 17: 85–95
5 DeMaria A, Vera Z, Amsterdam EA, Mason DT, Massumi RA (1974) Disturbances of cardiac rhythm and conduction induced by exercise. Diagnostic, prognostic and therapeutic implications. Am J Cardiol 33:732–736
6 Diamond GA, Forrester JS (1979) Analysis of prability as an aid in the clinical diagnosis of coronary-artery disease. N Engl J Med 300:1350–1358
7 Ellestad MH, Cooke BM Jr, Greenberg PS (1979) Stress testing: Clinical application and predictive capacity. Prog Cardiovasc Dis 21:431–460
8 Epstein SE (1979) Limitations of electrocardiographic exercise testing. N Engl J Med 301:264–265
9 Ericsson M, Granath A, Ahlsen P, Södermark T, Volpe U (1973) Arrhythmias and symptoms during treadmill testing three weeks after myocardial infarction. Br Heart J 35:787–790
10 Frick MH (1968) Coronary implications of hemodynamic changes caused by physical training. Am J Cardiol 22:417–425
11 Frick MH, Katile M (1968) Hemodynamic consequence of physical training after myocardial infarction. Circulation 37:192–202
12 Froelicher VF, Allen M, Lancaster M (1974) Maximal treadmill testing in normal USAF aircrewmen. Aeroscp Med 46:310–318
13 Goldschlager N, Cake D, Cohn K (1973) Exercise-induced ventricular arrhythmias in patients with coronary artery disease. Am J Cardiol 31:434–440

14 Goldschlager N, Cohn K, Goldschlager A (1979) Exercise-related ventricular arrhythmias. Mod Concepts Cardiovasc Dis 48:67–72
15 Helfant RH, Pine R, Kabde V, Banks VS (1974) Exercise-related ventricular premature complexes in coronary heart disease. Correlations with ischemia and angiographic severity. Ann Intern Med 80:589–592
16 Jackson G, Atkinson L, Oram S (1975) Reassessment of failed beta blocker treatment in angina pectoris by peak exercise heart rate measurements. Br Med J 3: 616–618
17 Kosowsky BD, Lown B, Whiting R, Guiney T (1971) Occurrence of ventricular arrhythmias with exercise as compared to monitoring. Circulation 44:826–832
18 Rifkin DR, Hood WB Jr (1977) Bayesian analysis of electrocardiographic exercise stress testing. N Engl J Med 297:681–686
19 Rochimis P, Blackburn H (1971) Exercise test: A survey of procedures, safety and litigation experience in approximately 170000 tests. JAMA 217:1061–1066
20 Ryan M, Lown B, Horn H (1975) Comparison of ventricular ectopic activity during 24-hour monitoring and exercise testing in patients with coronary heart disease. N Engl J Med 292:224–229
21 Sanne H (1973) Exercise tolerance and physical training of non-selected patients after myocardial infarction. Acta Med Scand (Suppl): 1–124
22 Sivarajan E, Snydsman AV, Smith B (1976) Feasibility study of low level treadmill testing for assessing acute myocardial infarction patients before discharge. Circulation (Suppl 2) 54:II–94
23 Smith JW, Denis CA, Gaines J, Gassmann A, Marcus FI, Staman M (1976) Activity evaluation test within three weeks after myocardial infarction. Circulation (Suppl 2) 54:II–10
24 Theroux P, Waters DD, Halphen C, Debaisieux J-G, Mizgala HF (1979) Prognostic value of exercise testing soon after myocardial infarction. N Engl J Med 301:341–345
25 Udall JA, Ellestad MH (1977) Predictive implications of ventricular premature contractions associated with treadmill stress testing. Circulation 56:985–989
26 Yasue H, Omote S, Takizawa A, Nagao M, Miwa K, Tanaka S (1979) Carcadian variation of exercise capacity in patients with Prinzmetal's variant angina: Role of exercise induced coronary arterial spasm. Circulation 59:938–948

Prognostic Value of Stress Testing

M.H. Ellestad

Introduction

The prognostic value of stress testing has a number of facets. Management of patients with ischemic heart disease requires a knowledge of the severity of anatomical obstruction to coronary flow and its effect on the myocardium at rest and during various exercise loads. It also requires a knowledge of how the ischemia effects the mechanics of performance of the heart and of the cardiac rhythmicity, and finally, how the peripheral mechanisms utilized by the body to adjust to the limited cardiac output interact. These mechanisms include the alterations in peripheral resistance and thus blood pressure responses, patterns of distribution such as skin blood flow responsible for heat loss, and also how the autonomic control of the heart rate reacts to various stresses. These immediate adjustments are of utmost importance in understanding how the patient responds to his environment, but it is also desirable to be able to predict the likelihood of future problems such as myocardial infarction and death. How well can we predict all these facets of cardiac behavior with stress testing?

Let us examine the various observations that can be made during stress testing and analyze how well they can serve our needs.

Electrocardiographic Changes

Only a few years ago the presence or absence of exercise-induced ST segment depression was the only observation reported and the final impression was labeled as positive or negative depending on the presence or absence of the ST response. Although ST segment depression is an important marker for ischemia, it represents only one of a number of parameters reflecting this process.

ST and EKG Contour

The contour of the ST segment is useful in predicting the severity of the disease process. The upsloping ST pattern presents a slightly lesser degree of ischemia than the horizontal, and the downsloping pattern usually denotes the most severe degree [21] (Fig. 1).

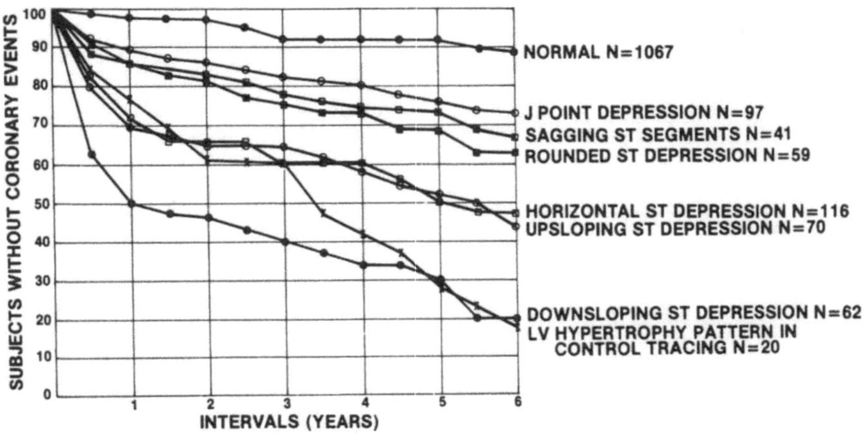

Fig. 1. Life table showing the combined coronary events incidence of all patterns

ST Elevation

Occasionally ST segment elevation rather than ST depression is induced by exercise. This change is probably produced by severe myocardial ischemia possibly involving the full thickness of the myocardium, inasmuch as 11 of 12 patients with this finding studied by Fortuin had total or near-total occlusion of a major coronary artery by angiography [13] (usually the LAD). Bartel [1] also found that patients with predominantly ST elevation during exercise were unlikely to have normal coronary arteriograms and consisted mainly of patients with disease of three coronary vessels. We [18] reported exercise-induced ST elevation in 14 of 29 patients (48%) with angiographically demonstrated left ventricular aneurysms, and failed to find these changes in the absence of left ventricular aneurysm in a consecutive list of 243 cases. It seems safe to say that ST elevation is consistent with an aneurysm if there is a known previous myocardial infarction, and if not, it consistently identifies high-grade ischemia [4], although this may be, at times, due to spasm [6].

R Wave Changes

Normal subjects have a reduction in precodial R wave amplitude with exercise after their heart rate exceeds about 120 [2]. Patients with coronary disease may have an increase in amplitude, often of 0.5 or more millivolts, apparently due to dilatation of the left ventricular volume as ischemia becomes manifested [3]. This change is proving useful in subjects without ST depression and also in evaluating patients with left bundle block. Work in our laboratory confirms that the changes in R wave amplitude reflect a volume change as measured by gated pool scintographic studies [12] (Fig. 2).

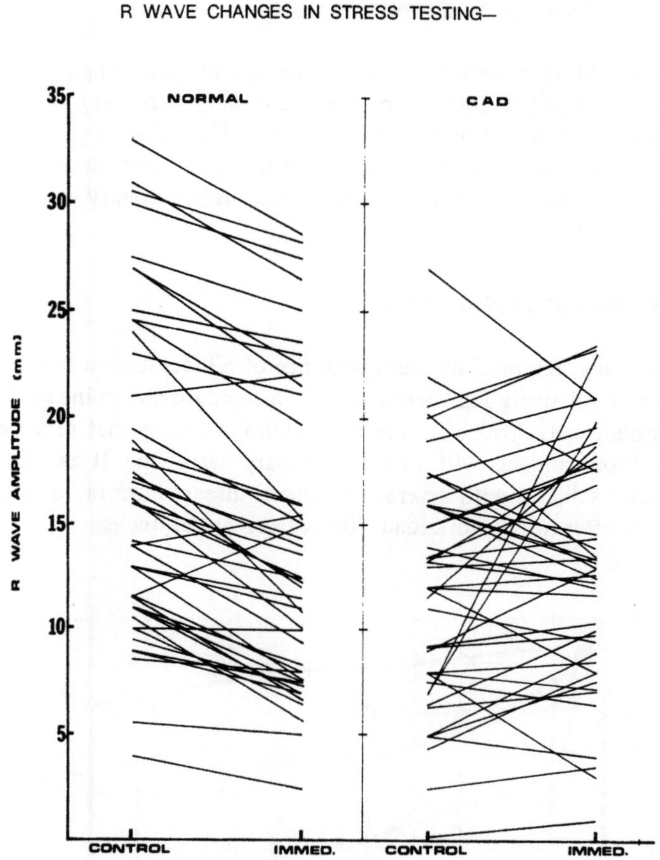

Fig. 2. Changes in *R wave* amplitude after exercise in subjects with normal coronary angiograms and in patients with coronary artery disease (CAD). *R wave* amplitude decreases in most of the normal subjects but increases in the subjects with coronary disease depending on the severity of the disease. Abbreviation: *IMMED*, immediate postexercise period

Magnitude of ST Depression

Although deep ST segment depression has always been associated with more ischemia than moderate changes, the magnitude of depression only emerges as a useful predictor when it is used after a light work load [8]. The more exercise necessary to cause the ST changes, the less value is the prediction drawn therefrom. We found that the magnitude of ST depression occuring with a light workload (4 METS) was very useful in predicting subsequent coronary events, while the magnitude of ST depression at higher work loads lost most of its specificity.

Time of Onset of ST Depression

As would be expected, ST depression manifested at light work loads or when the subjects is at rest denotes more severe coronary narrowing and is present when ischemia occurs with heavy or strenuous activity. Thus, during graded stress testing, ST depression early in the protocol not only denotes severy multivessel coronary disease, but also predicts a higher incidence of subsequent coronary events in the future (Fig. 3).

Duration of ST Depression

The time required for disappearance of ST depression during recovery is useful if one uses a relatively light work load or a standard end point for terminating exercise [14]. A high work load will produce metabolic effects that may persist for some time even in those subjects with limited coronary narrowing. It has also been demonstrated that many subjects with severe three-vessel disease have rapid resolution of ST depression, even after heavy work loads, for reasons as yet unclear.

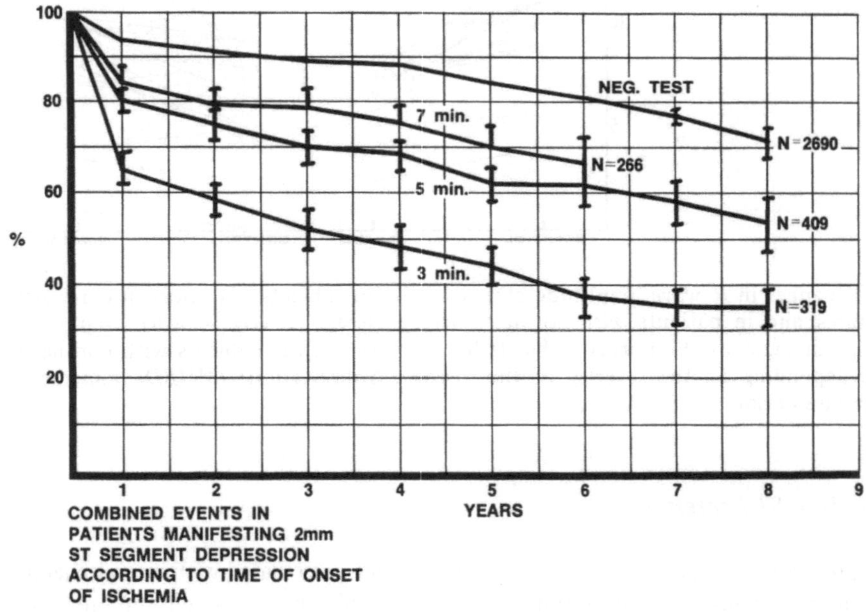

Fig. 3. Life table data depicting the incidence of coronary events according to the time of onset of severe ischemia during a maximum stress test. Note that in subjects with the onset of ischemia in the 3rd min (a work load of 4 mets), almost 65% had a coronary event by the 6th year

Blood Pressure Response

The failure of blood pressure to increase with exercise in a normal manner has been shown to prognosticate eventual coronary events and an inappropriate fall in blood pressure early in a graded testing protocol has been correlated with high-grade multivessel or left main disease [22]. The careful observation of these changes is also important in recognizing when or if the subject reaches his anaerobic threshold as well as in learning how his peripheral resistance responds to everyday exercise heart rate.

Heart Rate

It is now well documented [9, 17, 20] that an inappropriately low heart rate response, termed chronotropic incompetence, indicates decreased left ventricular function. We found it to be a reliable predictor of subsequent coronary events even in the absence of ST change. Many of these patients with inappropriate heart rate response also have the clinical syndrome of sick sinus syndrome.

Autonomic Response

The normal autonomic response to various maneuvers such as postural changes, cough, hyperventilation, and carotid massage have been shown to be altered in coronary disease. We have found that the blunting of a heart rate response to the first three of the above is predictive of significant coronary disease [15]. The usefulness of this type of data needs further evaluation, however.

Presence of Anginal Pain

When ischemic type ST changes are identified during stress testing, in the absence of anginal pain, a cohort of subjects with less severe disease is identified. The converse is true that when typical clinical angina occurs in conjunction with ST depression, the magnitude of disease is not only more severe, but denotes the likelihood of a higher incidence of significant coronary events in the immediate future [5]. There is no time better to evaluate the true nature of the angina of coronary insufficiency than during the time of an exercise test.

Exercise-Induced Arrhythmias

Numerous investigators have debated the importance of exercise-induced ventricular dysrhythmias in predicting coronary artery disease [16, 19]. In our study [23] of these changes, we found that those subjects with known coronary disease who also manifest ST depression have an added risk of subsequent coronary events, and should be viewed with this in mind. This is especially true when ventricular tachycardia occurs.

Multivariate Analysis and Likelihood Ratios

It stands to reason that the more data used to make a clinical decision, the more reliable will be the result. Thus, we have combined various findings in a multivariate computer program and found it to improve a diagnostic reliability [10]. We have also used the likelihood ratio proposed by Diamond and Forrester [7] to provide a percent probability of disease. In this way we have abandoned the concept of positive or negative stress tests for a statement describing the likelihood or posterior probability of disease. This type of information, we feel, is more in keeping with our knowledge of clinical events and should reduce the confusion surrounding the concepts of "false positives" or "false negatives" stress test.

The time has now arrived when the patient's ultimate outcome can be predicted more reliably by stress testing. Unless we consider the whole picture, however, such as the prevalence of disease in the patient being studied, the risk factors and their relationship to the individual patient and the clinical findings such as blood pressure, pain, and heart rate as well as the electrocardiographic changes, we will fall far short of the expectations of this useful procedure [11].

References

1 Bartel AG, Behar VS, Peter VS, Orgain ES, Long Y (1974) Graded exercise stress test in angiographically documented coronary artery disease. Circulation 49:348–356

2 Boronis PE, Greenberg PS, Christison GW, Castellanet MT, Ellestad MH (1978) Ability of R-wave amplitude (RWA) changes to reduce false negative (FN) and false positive (FP) responses by depression in treadmill stress testing (TST) (Abstract) Am J Cardiol 41:378

3 Bonoris PE, Greenberg PS, Christison GW et al. (1978) Evaluation of R wave amplitude changes versus ST segment depression in stress testing. Circulation 57: 904–910

4 Chahine RA, Raizher AE, Ishimori T (1976) The clinical significance of exercise-induced ST segment elevation. Circulation 54:209–213

5 Cole JP, Ellestad MH (1978) Significance of chest pain during treadmill exercise: Correlation with coronary events. Am J Cardiol 41:227–232

6 Detry JMR, Mengeot P, Rousseau MF, Cosyns J, Ponlot R, Brasseur LA (1975) Maximal exercise testing in patients with spontaneous angina pectoris associated with transient ST segment elevation. Risks and electrocardiographic findings. Br Heart J 37:897–903

7 Diamond GA, Forrester JS (1979) Analysis of probability as an aid in the clinical diagnosis of coronary artery disease. N Engl J Med 300:1350

8 Ellestad MH, Halliday WK (1977) Stress testing in the prognosis and management of ischemic heart disease. Angiology 28:149–159

9 Ellestad MH, Wan MKC (1975) Predictive implications of stress testing. Circulation 51:363–369

10 Ellestad MH, Savitz S, Bergdahl P, Teske J (1977) The false positive stress test: Multivariate analysis of 215 subjects with hemodynamic, angiographic, and clinical data. Am J Cardiol 40:681–685

11 Ellestad MH, Cooke BM, Greenberg PS (1979) Stress testing, clinical applications and predictive capacity. Prog Cardiovasc Dis 21:431

12 Ellestad MH, Greenberg PS, Berge R et al. (to be published) Comparison of R wave and ejection fraction changes during upright bicycle exercise: angiographic correlation. Yale J Biol Med
13 Fortuin NJ, Friesinger GC (1970) Exercise-induced ST segment elevation: Clinical, electrocardiographic and arteriographic studies in twelve patients. Am J Med 49: 459–464
14 Goldschlager N, Selzer A, Cohn K (1976) Treadmill stress tests as indicators of presence and severity of coronary artery disease. Ann Intern Med 85:277–286
15 Greenberg PS, Cooke BM Jr, Bible M, Ellestad MH (1980) Use of heart rate responses to standing and hyperventilation at rest to detect coronary artery disease: Correlation with the ST response to exercise. J Electrocardiology 13(4):373–378
16 Helfant RH, Pine R, Kabde V, Banka VS (1974) Exercise-related ventricular premature complexes in coronary heart disease. Ann Intern Med 80:589–592
17 Hinkle LE, Carver ST, Plakun A (1972) Slow heart rates and increased risk of cardiac death in middle aged men. Arch Intern Med 129:732–748
18 Manvi KN, Ellestad MH (1972) Elevated ST segments with exercise in ventricular aneurysm. J Electrocardioc 5:317–323
19 McHenry PL, Fisch C et al. (1972) Cardiac arrhythmias observed during maximal treadmill exercise testing in clinically normal men. Am J Cardiol 29:331–336
20 McNeer JF, Margolis JR, Lee KL, Kisslo JA, Peter RH, Kong Y, Behar MD, Wallace AG, McCants CB, Rosati RA (1978) The role of the exercise test in the evaluation of patients for ischemic heart disease. Circulation 57:64–70
21 Stuart RJ, Ellestad MH (1976) Upsloping ST segment in exercise stress testing. Am J Cardiol 37:19–22
22 Thompson PO, Keleman MH (1975) Hypotension accompanying the onset of exertional angina. Circulation 52:28–32
23 Udall JA, Ellestad MH (1977) Predictive implications of ventricular premature contractions associated with treadmill stress testing. Circulation 56:985–989

Part II
Coronary Angiography and Ventriculography

Methodology of Coronary Angiography and Ventriculography with Special Reference to Exercise

U. Gleichmann, G. Trieb, U. Sigwart, H. Mannebach, and D. Fassbender

Introduction

The technique of coronary and left ventricular angiography is well established and all cardiologists are familiar with it. *Coronary angiography* can be performed using the brachial cutdown technique of Sones or the percutaneous transfemoral method introduced by Judkins. There are no major differences in the rate of complications between these two techniques as shown by the last multicenter prospective cooperative study (CASS) published in 1979 [3]. The overall mortality rate was 2/1000, 1/1000 during the first 24 h and the other 1/1000 during the next 24 h, but none occurred in the catheter laboratory. The brachial procedure was associated with a higher risk of death, although this result is not found when analysis is restricted to laboratories with 80% or more brachial procedures. The risk of myocardial infarction (2.5/1000) was not significantly different for the two procedures. Prognostic factors increasing the risk of death were congestive heart failure, hypertension, left main coronary stenosis > 50%, an ejection fraction < 30%, and multiple premature ventricular contractions. Unstable angina increased the risk of myocardial infarction [3].

Left ventricular angiography is best done biplane in the right anterior oblique (RAO) position of 30°–40° and the left anterior oblique (LAO) position of 50°–60°. Left systolic (LVSP) and enddiastolic pressure (LVEDP), enddiastolic (EDVI) and endsystolic volume index (ESVI), and ejection fraction (EF) should be evaluated routinely using Dodge's area length [4] or Chapman's multiple slices method [2], with a calibration sphere exactly positioned at the site of the left ventricular cavity. This evaluation should be completed at least by a visual analysis of local wall motion. It is not the aim of this paper to give a detailed analysis of these techniques. There are many excellent papers and several excellent monographs on this topic [7, 10]. However, the interpretation of the results of coronary angiography may be difficult.

With the main topic of this symposium – the detection of ischemic myocardium with exercise – in mind, we want to concentrate on the clinical significance of coronary artery stenosis of various degrees and its correlation with left ventricular volume and pressure changes with exercise.

Significance of Coronary Stenosis

Nearly all reports on coronary angiograms and their relation to treatment and prognosis use poorly defined groups of coronary stenosis expressed in percent stenosis. More recently a grading system was introduced which was proposed first by Gensini and later by an ad hoc committee under the auspices of the American Heart Association [7]. This system lists a scale of lumen diameter reduction of a vessel by 25%, 50%, 75%, 99%, and 100% stenoses (Fig. 1). Stenoses of less than 50% are most often accepted as insignificant at rest and with exercise, of more than 90% as critical [11, 15]. This is in agreement with the experimental data of Gould et al. [8], which indicate that the capacity to increase the coronary flow significantly in response to additional oxygen demands is abolished when there is an 88%–93% diameter constriction, just after resting flow begins to diminish. At this point all compensatory mechanisms are exhausted at rest.

Problems arise in the interpretation of the functional significance of moderate stenosis of 50%–75%. From experimental data [8] we know that this degree of stenosis can be partially compensated for by a reduction in peripheral coronary resistance which is in series with a proximal stenosis. Paulin [11] has indicated that this mechanism readily explains the frequent observations made in clinical coronary angiography that an apparent, very narrow stenosis may be present without resulting in a demonstrable delay in peripheral contrast filling. On the other hand, an increase in oxygen demand of the myocardium or a small increase in the percentage of stenosis due to coronary artery spasm or thrombosis may suddenly decrease coronary artery flow in this type of moderate stenosis. After finishing exercise ventriculography we have observed coronary artery spasm in patients with minor or moderate coronary stenosis and normal ventricular function at rest and with exercise. This could explain the observation that in some patients angina pectoris does not occur during but rather shortly after exercise. The functional significance of this moderate stenosis depends furthermore on the area and thickness of the perfused muscle and is influenced by perfusion pressure, myocardial oxygen consumption, and collateral flow between this area and other parts of the ventricle. With these variables in mind, one must conclude that the critical lumen diameter reduction lies somewhere

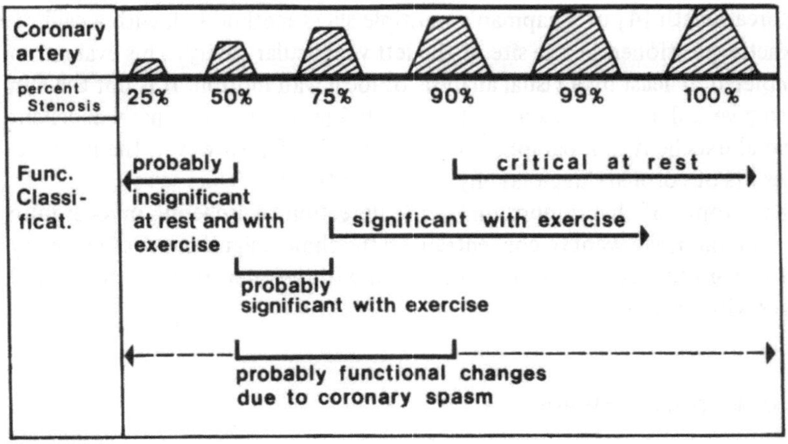

Fig. 1. Grading system of coronary stenosis in percent diameter reduction and significance of coronary stensosis in coronary heart disease

between 50% and 90% stenosis and that it must be impossible to define a sharp borderline between significant and insignificant stenosis for an individual patient. A higher angiographic resolution would not resolve this problem. The intercorrelation of these parameters for an individual patient and the prediction of the extent of myocardium in jeopardy in a given patient prior to myocardial infarction could only be determined experimentally with exercise and by analyzing local wall motion with exercise angiography [5, 6, 12, 13, 14, 16, 17] or with perfusion scintigraphy [1].

Ventricular Volume and Pressure Changes During Exercise

It is surprising that only a few of us would consider it necessary to look at left ventricular volumes and ejection fraction during exercise despite the fact that most coronary patients develop problems during exertion. In our experience, left ventricular angiography during exercise is a safe and effective method of improving diagnostic accuracy of coronary angiography. So we would like to make some technical comments regarding the method and present some results of the correlation of left ventricular function with various degrees and locations of coronary stenosis.

Method

Catheters were introduced in most cases by the Judkins technique and in a small group of 5% by the Sones technique. The introduction through the right or left groin does not interfere with the bicycle exercise in any way. Before exercise, measurements of pressure and cardiac output (using thermodilution technique) and biplane left ventriculography were performed at rest. The resting left ventricular angiogram was obtained with power injections of approximately 0.5–0.6 ml/kg Urografin 76 with a flow rate of 12 ml/s; for the exercise left ventricular angiogram a slightly higher quantity of 0.6–0.7 ml/kg and a higher flow rate of 14–16 ml/s were chosen. For the exercise ventriculogram the patient was asked to continue the effort on the electrically braked bicycle ergometer in the supine position. Mild inspiration was assured during injection. Cineangiograms in the RAO 30° and LAO 60° positions were obtained simultaneously at a film speed of 50 frames per second. The work load used depended on the patient's history, preceding noninvasive or semi-invasive studies using ECG at rest and with exercise, echocardiography, and pulmonary artery pressure measurements made with a floating catheter. The mean work load was 52 W with a range of 30–80 W.

Angiography was performed during exercise when heart rate increased to approximately 110 beats/min or LVEDP increased to more than 40 mm Hg or the patient reported angina pectoris. Using these end points exercise was submaximal in most patients. Selective coronary angiography was performed 5–10 min after stopping exercise. Thus the time for the entire catherization procedure was 40–60 min. With the experience of some 750 exercise ventriculographies we now prefer coronary angiography before ventriculography, which provides the advantage of knowing the patient's coronary state. A delay of 10 min is considered sufficient to negate the hemodynamic effects of the contrast medium. Although higher heart rates are desirable from a physiologic standpoint, the lack of adequate opacification due to rapid washout of contrast medium renders them impractical.

More than 750 patients have been studied since 1975 – about 25% of all the catheterizations conducted. There were no complications at the site of catheter entrance or due to contrast injections which could be attributed to the exercise procedure. There were extrasystoles in 12% of patients at rest and in 11% with exercise. Mean heart rate increased from 72 to 104 beats/min for the evaluation of the results. Coronary stenosis was graded according to Gensini [7]. Analysis of the ventriculogram was performed according to the biplane area length method of Dodge using a viodeometric device.

Results

Only our results in normals and in patients with 75% or higher stenosis without myocardial infarction have been used to draw general conclusions.

Normal Reaction

About 130 subjects were assumed to be normal (Table 1). In other words, no evidence of any organic heart disease could be detected. In this group the resting heart rate increased from 75 to 108 beats/min, systolic pressure from 130 to 158 mm Hg, left ventricular enddiastolic pressure from 9.5 to 20 mm Hg, and EDVI from 74 to 80 with unchanged ESVI, and there was a small increase in ejection fraction from 65% to 68%. Cardiac index (CI) increased from 2.9 to 4.7 liter/m^2. In single circumflex (CX) or right coronary artery (RCA) stenosis there was nearly the same increase in heart rate, LVSP, EDVI, and CI with unchanged ESVI and EF but an abnormal increase in the LVEDP from 15 to 32 mm Hg (Table 2). Thus, pump function remained unchanged with a higher filling pressure. The diminished contraction of the posterior wall is compensated for by an increased contraction pattern of the normally perfused anterior wall.

Also very interesting are the findings in single left anterior descending artery (LAD) stenosis of 50% compared with 75% stenosis with and without angina pectoris during exercise (Fig. 2). Compared to normals, in 50% LAD stenosis there was a slight increase in LVEDP and mean PAP, but a normal increase in CI and EDVI, and a slight decrease in ESVI such that EF increased as in normals. Thus, in isolated 50% LAD stenosis all volume parameters under exercise did not behave significantly differently from normals with a small increased filling pressure. Perhaps with more sophisticated methods it will be possible to demonstrate local wall motion disorders in 50% stenosis, too.

This is true for 75% stenosis without angina pectoris in which EDVI and ESVI increased to the same amount, so that EF did not increase but remained unchanged. In the 75% LAD stenosis with angina pectoris during exercise the greatest increase was in LVEDP, EDVI, and ESVI resulting in a drop in EF. But in spite of this decreased EF, CI remained increased, though on a somewhat lower level compared to the other groups. In two- or three-vessel disease involving the LAD we most often found changes similar to, or more pronounced than in 75% LAD stenosis with angina pectoris with exercise (Table 3).

Table 1. Hemodynamic parameters at rest and during exercise in normals (mean and SD); *n*, 137

Parameters	Rest	Exercise	Δ
HR	74.9	108.4	+ 33.5
(beats/min)	± 11	± 17	
LVSP	130.8	154.9	+ 24.1
(mmHg)	± 16	± 20	
LVEDP	9.5	20.2	+ 10.7
(mmHg)	± 4	± 4	
EDVI	73.7	79.8	+ 6.1
(ml/m^2)	± 18	± 22	
ESVI	26.6	26.1	- 0.5
(ml/m^2)	± 15	± 16	
EF	65.0	68.2	+ 3.2
(%)	± 11	± 11	
CI	2.96	4.72	+ 1.76
$(l/min/m^2)$	± 0.6	± 1.1	+ 1.76

Table 2. Hemodynamic parameters at rest and during exercise (mean and SD) in isolated stenosis of right coronary artery or circumflex branch of left coronary artery; *n*, 10

Parameters	Rest	Exercise	Δ
HR	66.5	94.5	+ 28.0
(beats/min)	± 13	± 15	
LVSP	131.7	156.3	+ 24.6
(mmHg)	± 9	± 23	
LVEDP	12.4	26.6	+ 14.2
(ml/m^2)	± 6	± 5	
EDVI	73.7	81.0	+ 7.3
(ml/m^2)	± 12	± 12	
ESVI	28.2	28.1	- 0.1
(ml/m^2)	± 12	± 17	
EF	64.3	64.9	+ 0.6
(%)	± 8	± 8	
CI	3.02	4.45	+ 1.43
$(l/min/m^2)$	± 0.6	± 1.1	

Using the above-mentioned protocol, exercise was discontinued due to symptoms in only about 25% of the patients studied. In most cases exercise was stopped at a heart rate of not more than 110 beats/min to achieve satisfactory opacification of exercise angiography. This enabled us to analyze the sequence of appearance of abnormal hemodynamic parameters from a synthesis of the results of many tests. During the first phase of ischemia there is an increase in filling pressure without significant changes in volume parameters (Fig. 3). Enddiastolic volume and endsystolic volume increase by the same degree so that the ejection fraction remains constant. With angina pectoris there is a sudden drop in EF but CI remains unchanged up to this point. How-

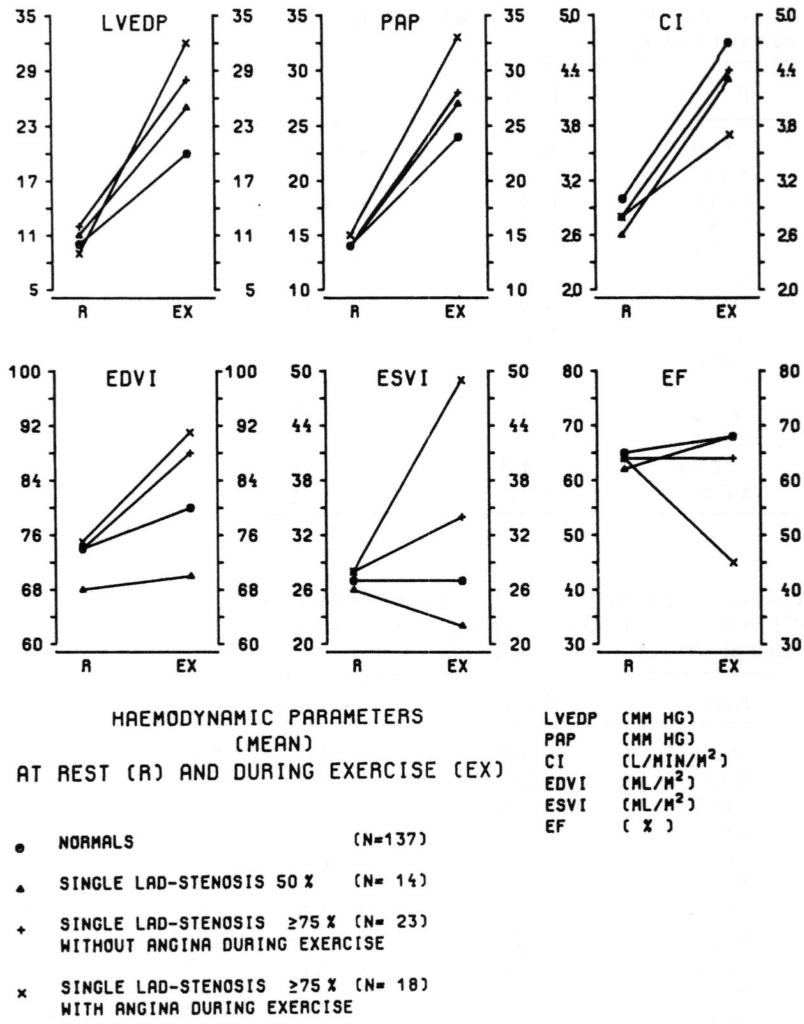

Fig. 2. Volume and pressure changes in different degrees of left anterior descending (*LAD*) stenosis

ever, with a further increase of ischemia, a further decrease in EF and finally of CI could be observed.

Not only the degree of stenosis, but also the extent and the position of the ischemic wall segment distal to the stenosis, influence left ventricular pump function to various degrees during exercise (Fig. 4). Anterior wall ischemia appears to have a greater impact on ventricular function than inferior or posterior wall ischemia. From our results we can summarize as follows: the lowest level of ischemia appears to cause mainly compliance disturbances (Figs. 2, 3). At this level, the overall contractile behavior might still be unchanged, but mild ST changes may appear. A higher level of ischemia seems to cause contractile disturbances starting with regional wall motion disorders such as retarded contraction of one or two segments. If a posterior wall ischemia comprises

Table 3. Hemodynamic parameters (mean and SD) at rest and during exercise in three-vessel disease of left main stenosis; *n*, 19

Parameters	Rest	Exercise	Δ
HR	70.4	103.2	+ 32.8
(beats/min)	± 10	± 14	
LVSP	138.8	152.9	+ 14.1
(mmHg)	± 16	± 20	
LVEDP	10.8	31.1	+ 20.3
(mmHg)	± 3	± 9	
EDVI	73.5	83.4	+ 9.9
(ml/m^2)	± 20	± 24	
ESVI	27.8	39.8	+ 12.0
(ml/m^2)	± 11	± 20	
EF	61.9	54.3	- 7.6
(%)	± 10	± 14	
CI	2.59	4.12	1.53
($l/min/m^2$)	± 0.5	± 12	

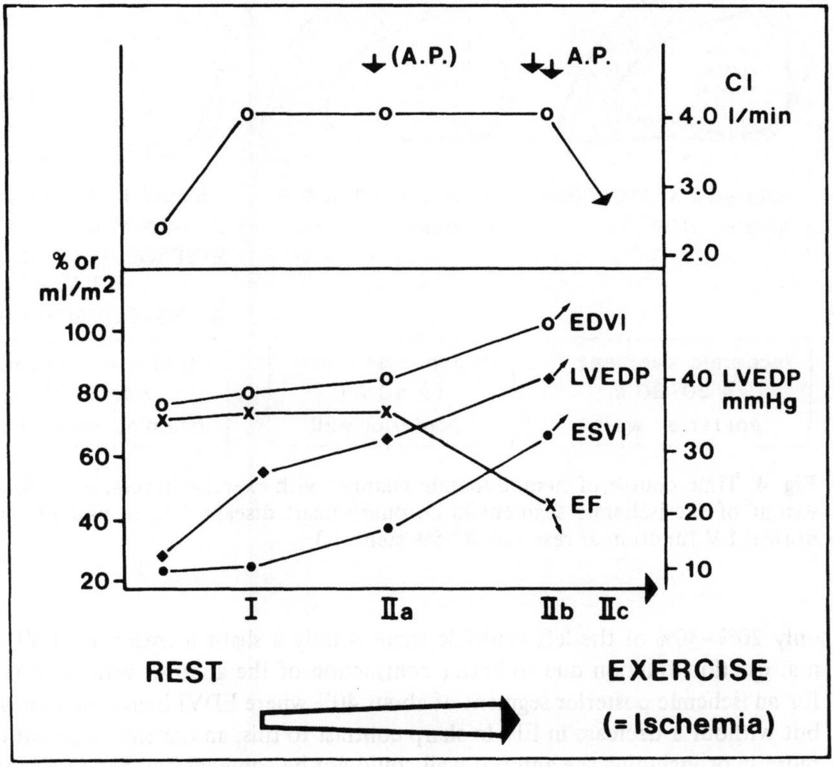

Fig. 3. Time course of volume and pressure changes during exercise in CHD (single LAD two- or three-vessel disease ≥ 75% stenosis)

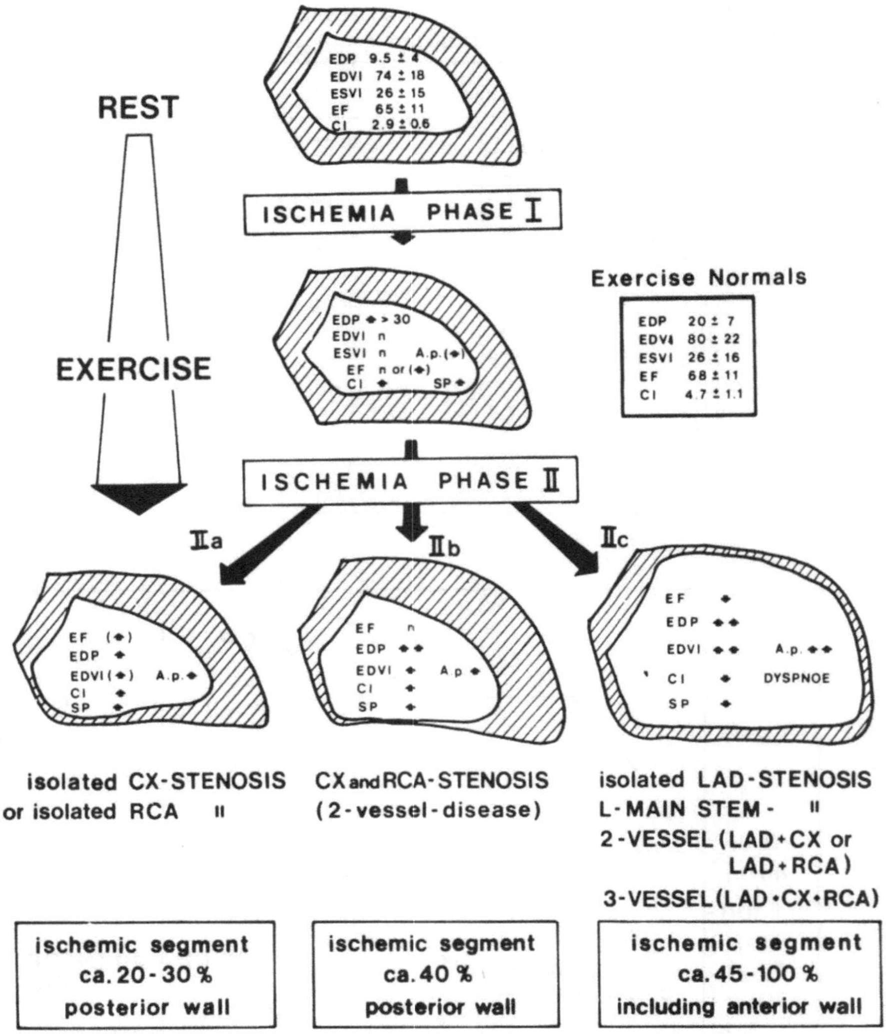

Fig. 4. Time course of hemodynamic changes with exercise in relation to location and extent of the ischemic segment in coronary heart disease, i.e., in patients with CHD, normal LV function at rest and ⩾ 75% stenosis)

only 20%–30% of the left ventricle there is only a slight increase in EDVI, with normal ejection fraction due to better contraction of the anterior wall. This is also true for an ischemic posterior segment of about 40% where EDVI increases somewhat more but without a decrease in EF. In sharp contrast to this, an ischemic segment of 45% or more in or including the anterior wall could not be compensated for by better contraction of the posterior wall; so EF and CI decrease.

In summary a correlation exists between coronary anatomy and pathophysiology in coronary heart disease [9]. In cases with normal resting LV function this correlation is optimally demonstrated with exercise ventriculography, which has been shown to be a

Table 4. Indications for left ventricular angiography during exercise in patients

In normal or nearly normal LV function at rest:

1. In CHD (one-vessel disease):
   a) Significance of LAD stensosis on left ventricular function in cases with healed small myocardial infarction or without myocardial infarction (predicting the extend of myocardium in jeopardy)
   b) LV function in segmental early relaxation
2. In CHD (two- or three-vessel disease):
   a) Overall left ventricular function with exercise
   b) Functional significance of LAD stenosis
3. Without CHD
   a) LV function with exercise in cases with angina pectoris
   b) LV function with exercise in cases with abnormal ST changes

In abnormal LV function at rest:

1. In CHD:
   a) Function of ventricle in cases with aneurysm of left anterior wall
2. Without CHD:
   b) Detection of a so-called lazy ventricle
   (abnormal EF at rest, normalization of EF with exercise)

safe and effective procedure when used routinely. The present indications for left ventriculography during exercise are given in Table 4. The correlation between organic lesions and physiology is most obvious in the presence of LAD stenosis. A stenosis of 50%–60% in a dominant LAD should be regarded as significant. The same degree of lesion in the circumflex or right coronary artery alone may well be accompanied by a compensatory hypercontractility of the anterior wall.

Summary

The technique of coronary and left ventricular angiography is well established and all cardiologists are familiar with it. There are no major differences in risk or complications between the Sones and Judkins techniques. However, the interpretation of the results of coronary angiography may be difficult. Stenosis of less than 50% diameter is generally accepted as insignificant; stenosis of more than 90% is seen as critical.

Problems arise in the interpretation of the functional significance of moderate stenosis between 50% and 70%, especially in the left anterior descending artery. This degree of stenosis could be partially compensated for by a reduction of peripheral coronary resistance. On the other hand, coronary spasm could suddenly increase a moderate stenosis. The functional significance of this degree of stenosis is further influenced by perfusion pressure and myocardial oxygen consumption.

Left ventriculography during supine exercise is one method of further evaluating stenoses that are moderate to critical in degree, and of predicting the extent of myocardium in jeopardy in a given patient prior to myocardial infarction. From our experience with 730 exercise ventriculograms the following conclusions can be drawn. Phase 1: In mild exercise-induced ischemia, 75% stenosis, and normal function at rest, a compliance disorder with increasing enddiastolic pressure (EDP) develops without altered regional mechanical myocardial performance. Ejection fraction (EF) increases or remains unchanged, enddiastolic volume index (EDVI) is normal, and cardiac index (CI) is increased. Phase 2 of ischemia shows local hypokinesia or akinesia with increasing EDVI and an unchanged EF and CI in cases with posterior wall ischemia (CX and/or RCA stensosis) and normal anterior wall, which compensates for posterior wall dyskinesia. However, in anterior and/or lateral wall ischemia (isolated LAD, LAD + CX, left main stenosis) there is a marked increase in EDP and EDVI with a decrease in EF and, finally, CI. In 50% stenosis of the LAD, no local wall motion disorders could be detected during exercise in spite of an increase in EDP.

On the other hand, left ventricular exercise angiography in patients with syndrom X (angina pectoris, normal coronary arteries) could be applied for differentiating between compliance and/or pump function disorders.

References

1 Borer JS, Bacharach SL, Green MV, Kent KM, Epstein SE, Johnson GS (1977) Realtime radionuclide cineangiography in the noninvasive evaluation of global and regional left ventricular function at rest and with exercise in patients with coronary heart disease. N Engl J Med 296:839

2 Chapman CB, Baker O, Reynolds H, Bonke FJ (1958) Use of biplane cinefluorography for measurement of ventricular volume. Circulation 18:1105

3 Davis K, Kennedy JW, Kemp HG, Judkins P, Gosselin A, Killip T (1979) Complications of coronary arteriography from the collaborative study of coronary artery surgery (CASS). Circulation 59:1105

4 Dodge HT, Sandler H, Baxley WH, Hawley RR (1966) Usefullness and limitations of radiographic methods for determing left ventricular volume. Am J Cardiol 18:10

5 Eubanks DE, Tsakiris AG, Davis GD, Wallace RB, Frye RL (1970) Left ventricular volumes during exercise induced angina in patients with coronary artery disease. Circulation (Suppl III) 41–42:151

6 Frischknecht J, Steele P, Kirch D, Jensen D, Vogel R (1979) Effect of exercise on left ventricular ejection fraction in men with coronary artery disease. Am Heart J 97:494

7 Gensini GG (1975) Coronary-Arteriography. Vol. 33. Futura, New York, pp 87–94

8 Gould L, Lipscomb K, Hamiltin G (1974) Physiologic basis for assessing critical coronary stenosis. Am J Cardiol 33:87–94

9 Iskandrian AS, Segal BL (1979) Structure and function of the coronary arteries: How are they related? Cathet Cardiovasc Diagn 5:101–105

10 Lichtlen P (1979) Koronarangiographie. Dr. med. D. Straube Verlag, Erlangen

11 Paulin S (1979) Gradin and measering coronary artery stenoses. Cathet Cardiovasc Diagn 5:213–218

12 Sharman B, Goodwin JF, Raphael MJ, Steiner RE, Rainbow RG, Taylor SH (1976) Left ventricular angiography on exercise: A new method of assessing left ventricular function in ischemic heart disease. Br Heart J 38:59

13 Sigwart U, Schmidt H, Bonzel T, Mertens HM, Gleichmann U (1975) Biplane cineangiographic evaluation of left ventricular concentration in ischemic heart disease at rest and during bicycle exercise. Circulation (Suppl II) 51:37

14 Sigwart U, Schmidt H, Steiner J, Mertens HM, Gleichmann U (1975) Linksventrikuläre Geometrie und Volumina in Ruhe und während Ergometerbelastung bei koronarer Herzkrankheit. Verh Dtsch Ges Kreislaufforsch 41:193

15 Swan HJ (1979) Mechanical function of the heart and its alteration during myocardial ischemia and infarction. Circulation 60/7:1587
16 Trieb G, Sigwart U, Mannebach H, Mertens HM, Gleichmann U (1979) Evaluation of left-ventricular disfunction in coronary heart-disease by pressure, flow and volume parameters during stress. Z Kardiol 68/4:260
17 Trieb G, Sigwart U, Mannebach H, Mertens HM, Gleichmann U (to be published) Left ventricular volume and ejection fraction during supine exercise in patients with and without heart disease. Cardiology

Relationship Between Coronary Obstructions and Regional Myocardial Blood Flow in Man During Stress Provoked by Rapid Atrial Pacing

P.R. Lichtlen and H.J. Engel

Introduction

Today's knowledge of the behavior of coronary flow in poststenotic myocardial regions during increased oxygen demand is based mainly on results from acute animal experiments [5, 12, 16, 20, 22]. They correlate flow to the degree of obstruction by reducing stepwise the diameter of large extramural coronary arteries, and in addition, analyze coronary reserve, i.e., flow during maximal arteriolar dilation induced by reactive hyperemia. Thus, it was demonstrated [6, 7] that at rest mean coronary flow is only impaired at a diameter reduction of 85%, whereas the limitation of coronary reserve, i.e., of flow during hyperemic response, has already begun at a diameter reduction of 45% and is completely abolished at 93%. Hence, from this and other studies [16, 20], it would appear that also in man at rest poststenotic flow should remain unaltered up to obstructions of at least 75% and that during maximal flow, exhibited during any form of stress, a proximal, fixed coronary obstruction would begin to influence flow at a much lesser degree of stenosis, i.e., at approximately 50%.

For the situation at rest, this concept was by and large verified in patients with severe coronary disease [4, 11, 14]. Poststenotic flow was found to be normal even with obstructions of 90% or more as long as left ventricular (LV) wall motion remained unaltered; it decreased, however, in accordance with the impairment of poststenotic LV wall motion. On the other hand, only a few investigations exist on the behavior of coronary flow during stress in patients with high-degree coronary obstructions [2, 3, 8, 9, 10, 15, 21]. This is due to several reasons: first, in man, regional myocardial blood flow, i.e., coronary flow in the ischemic area is technically difficult to assess during any type of stress. It necessitates the use of gamma cameras, which alone enable the spatial separation of normal and poststenotic areas in the same heart. Not only the size of the camera, but especially as yet unsolved theoretical and practical problems ("smear effects" during fast heart rates, geometric changes due to heavy breathing, etc.) render their use during bicycle ergometry almost impossible. Therefore, most studies so far have concentrated on the registration of global myocardial blood flow [3, 8, 9, 10], recording flow from the entire heart by a small single scintillation probe, including normal and abnormal areas. This technique, however, can only partially reflect the behavior of flow in poststenotic regions, as the washout curve of the isotope mainly reflects the fast component, i.e., flow from the normal area [13, 14]. Hence, only very few studies have made use of the regional technique so far [2, 15, 21], all provoking stress by rapid atrial pacing.

Second, the exact measurement of coronary obstructions from cineangiograms is still difficult, time consuming, and in many regards, unsatisfactory (problem of measuring accurately small distances (less than 2 mm) from the angiogram); nevertheless, we feel that today the degree of accuracy allows fairly exact measurements of coronary obstructions [17, 18], these values being by far more reliable than those obtained from estimates.

It is therefore the aim of this study to analyze regional myocardial blood flow during pacing-induced ischemia by comparing, for the first time, poststenotic and normal flow in the same patient and relating flow to the quantitated degree of obstruction.

Methods

Patients

Regional myocardial blood flow (RMBF) was studied at rest and during ischemia provoked by rapid right atrial pacing (RAP) in 28 coronary patients, mean age 51 years, all undergoing selective coronary and left ventricular angiography 1 h prior to the study. All patients had severe angina and demonstrated typical ST depressions ($\geqslant$ 0.2 mV) during bicycle ergometry performed the day before the flow study. In addition, coronary angiography had to reveal one high-grade isolated obstruction of the left anterior descending (LAD), the left circumflex branch (LCX), or the right coronary artery (RCA), the obstructions ranging between 52% and 100% (Table 1). In order to be able to compare flow from the poststenotic area with a normal area, patients with multiple obstructions or triple vessel disease were excluded from the study. Finally, coronary obstructions were quantitated from cineangiograms (see below). Thus, RMBF was registered and compared in the poststenotic and the normal area of each patient with the aid of the regional precordial Xenon clearance technique. Fifteen minutes after the assessment of control (resting, flow, right atrial pacing averaging 142 beats/min was instituted and coronary flow was registered during 2 min following angina and/or St depressions of more than 0.1 mV.

Assessment of Coronary Obstructions

Coronary obstructions were measured from coronary angiograms (35-mm cine films, 32 frames) taken in various projections: left anterior oblique (LAO) 40%, posterior-anterior (PA), right anterior oblique (RAO) 30° and 60° (right and left half axials) employing a vernier with an accuracy of 0.05 mm, the tip of the catheter (Judkins catheter, average 1.8 mm) being used for calibration. Measurements of the diameter of the coronary arteries were done shortly above the obstruction, at the widest point, and within the obstruction, i.e., at the narrowest point. Calculations of the degree of obstruction were based on average measurements from several projections, the following formula being used:

$$\% \text{ stenosis (area)} = \left[1 - \frac{D_{\text{sten}}{}^2}{D_{\text{presten}}{}^2}\right] \cdot 100$$

where D_{sten} corresponds to the narrowest diameter with stenosis and D_{presten} to the largest diameter above the stenosis [17].

Table 1. Regional myocardial blood flow under ischemia provoked by right atrial pacing (n = 28)

	Obstructed artery (poststenotic area)			
Degree of Obstruction	LAD	LCX	RCA	Total
100% (collaterals)	11	–	2	13
91%–99%	1 (95%)	–	–	1 (95%)
⩽ 90%	9 (71.1.%)	5 (77.6%)	–	14 (73.4%)
	21 (87.4%)	5 (77.6%)	2 (100%)	28 86.5%)

Normal zone: LCX n = 21
LAD n = 7

Table 1 demonstrates the distribution of coronary obstructions in the 28 patients. In 21 cases (87%), the obstruction was located in the proximal LAD; 11 times a total occlusion was present, and the middle and distal parts of the LAD were filled by large collaterals originating from the RCA. In ten cases, coronary flow of the LAD occurred still in an antegrade way, the degree of obstruction being once above 90%, and nine times 90% or less, averaging 71% (52%–90%). Five times the obstructions concerned the left circumflex branch and were below 90%, averaging 77% (75%–83%). A complete obstruction of the RCA was present twice, the distal branches being filled by collaterals originating from the left circumflex branch and/or the LAD. Altogether the obstructions averaged 86.5% cross sectional area. The normal area, i.e., the myocardial zone perfused by normal or only mildly stenosed vessels (obstructions less than 30%) – that is the region used to record control flow – belonged 21 times to the left circumflex and seven times to the left anterior descending branch.

Left Ventricular Wall Motion

Left ventricular wall motion was assessed from left ventricular angiograms taken in 40° RAO projection (injection of 35 ml Urografin 65%) and at 80 frames. Wall motion was determined from six halfaxes drawn perpendicularly on the longitudinal axis (aortic-mitral valve junction to the apex) in 25% distances; this resulted in three superior and three inferior axes. Percent systolic shortening was measured from end-systolic and enddiastolic silhouettes of the left ventricular angiogram and shortening was regarded as normal above 25% (normokinesis), as hypokinetic between 10% and 25%, and as akinetic below 10% (for details see [26]). Table 2 summarizes the relationship between poststenotic wall motion and the degree and location of coronary obstructions. Left ventricular wall motion of the poststenotic area was 11 times normokinetic, 8 times hypokinetic and 9 times akinetic. In all of the latter nine patients, the akinetic region, i.e., the infarct, was small and located in the apical area, proximal to

Table 2. LV wall motion in relation to degree of obstruction

LV wall motion	LAD 100%	LAD 99%–91%	LAD ⩽90%	LCX ⩽90%	RCA 100%	Total
Normokinetic (SS > 25%)	2	1	4	3	1	11
Hypokinetic (SS 10%–25%)	4	–	3	1		8
Akinetic	5	–	2	1	1	9
(SS < 10%)	5	–	2	1	1	9
	11	1	9	5	2	28
		21				

the papillary muscles. Patients with large infarctions comprising more than 20% of the circumferential area of the left ventricular angiogram, were excluded from the study.

Assessment of Regional Myocardial Blood Flow by the Precordial Xenon Clearance Technique

Coronary flow was measured with the aid of the precordial regional Xenon clearance technique (for details see [11]). Under fluoroscopic control 10–20 mCi Xenon 133 was injected into the main left coronary artery. The patient was then immediately moved under the gamma camera, which was set at an LAO projection of 40° in order to separate the region perfused by the LAD from the one of the LCX. A pho gamma III camera (Nuclear Chicago), connected to a CDC 1700 computer system, was used for flow recording (deadtime of the system 4 μs). During the first 60 s of washout, the the frame length was 2 s; during the second 60 s, it was 5 s. Calculation of washout followed the Kety-Schmidt formula; the first 30 s were regarded as monoexponential. Flow was calculated for each matrix point, approximately 400–600 matrix points covering the heart; in addition, larger areas of 25 matrix points and – according to the angiographic aspect of each patient – regions perfused by the LAD, LCX, and distal RCA – were defined.

Flow was displayed both numerically (ml/min per 100 g myocardium) as well as in an analog fashion as "flow scan," i.e., a functional image indicating the different levels of flow for each matrix point in various colors. Certain statistics were applied excluding falsely low counts, i.e., statistically unacceptable washout curves as well as extracardiac counts [11].

Results

Regional Myocardial Blood Flow in the Poststenotic Zone During Ischemia

Figure 1 shows a typical example of a flow measurement at rest and during ischemia provoked by rapid atrial pacing, before and after nitroglycerin, in a patient with isolated (> 90%) obstruction of the LAD. At rest, flow in the poststenotic zone of the LAD amounted to 56 ml/min per 100 g myocardium, in the normal area of the LCX, it was, at 60 ml/min per 100 g, somewhat higher. Pacing up to 130 beats/min led to angina and typical ST depressions; in the poststenotic zone, flow remained unchanged with 60 ml/min per 100 g; in the normal area, it increased to 90 ml/min per 100 g (+ 50%). It must be assumed that flow in the normal zone corresponded to the actual myocardial oxygen consumption for this level of pacing; this would indicate a marked flow deficit in the poststenotic zone. The second period of pacing after 0.8 mg nitroglycerin sublingually shows decreased, but now equal flow levels both in the normal and poststenotic zone. Angina and ST depressions were absent at this time.

Figure 2 summarizes the changes in RMBF in all 28 cases, regardless of the degree of obstruction. During right atrial pacing, the rate pressure product (RPP) increased from 94 to 175 mm Hg $\cdot$ min^{-1} $\cdot$ 10^{-2} ($P < 0.01$), mainly due to the increase in heart rate from an average of 73 to 142 beats/min; the systolic pressure remaining unchanged with 127 and 124 mm Hg, respectively. Thus, according to the RPP, myocardial oxygen consumption increased by approximately 86%. At rest, RMBF was at 56 ml/min per 100 g significantly lower in the poststenotic than in the normal area where it averaged 68 ml/min per 100 g ($P < 0.0005$), a phenomenon which was described earlier by our group [11, 14]. During rapid atrial pacing (RAP), RMBF increased significantly both in the normal area (+ 28 ml/min per 100 g; + 42.5%; $P < 0.0005$) as well as in the poststenotic zone (+ 22 ml/min per 100 g; + 37.8%; $P < 0.0005$). However. this incrase reached at 95 ml/min per 100 g significantly higher level in the normal area than in the poststenotic zone with 78 ml/min per 100 g ($P < 0.0005$).

Thus, in patients with severe coronary artery disease, stress-induced angina pectoris and ST depressions are associated with an insufficient increase in transmural RMBF in the poststenotic zone. As flow of the poststenotic and normal area was simultaneously registered in each patient, it seems reasonable to assume that RMBF in the normal area corresponded to the oxygen demand for this RPP, i.e., the actual level of oxygen demand; thus, flow in the poststenotic zone represented a marked deficit of oxygen delivery.

Poststenotic Flow During Ischemia in Relation to the Degree of Obstruction

Figure 3 demonstrates the behavior of flow in poststenotic areas perfused by coronary arteries with obstructions of ⩽ 90% and > 90%, i.e., total occlusion and retrograde collateral filling, mainly of the LAD (11 patients) or the distal RCA (two cases). In patients with obstructions ⩽ 90%, heart rate was increased from 70 to 141 beats/min, and in patients with obstructions above 90% from 75 to 143 beats/min; also the average RPP reached during pacing in the two groups did not differ significantly (179 and 171 mm Hg per min^{-1} $\cdot$ 10^{-2}, respectively). Resting flow was equal in the post-

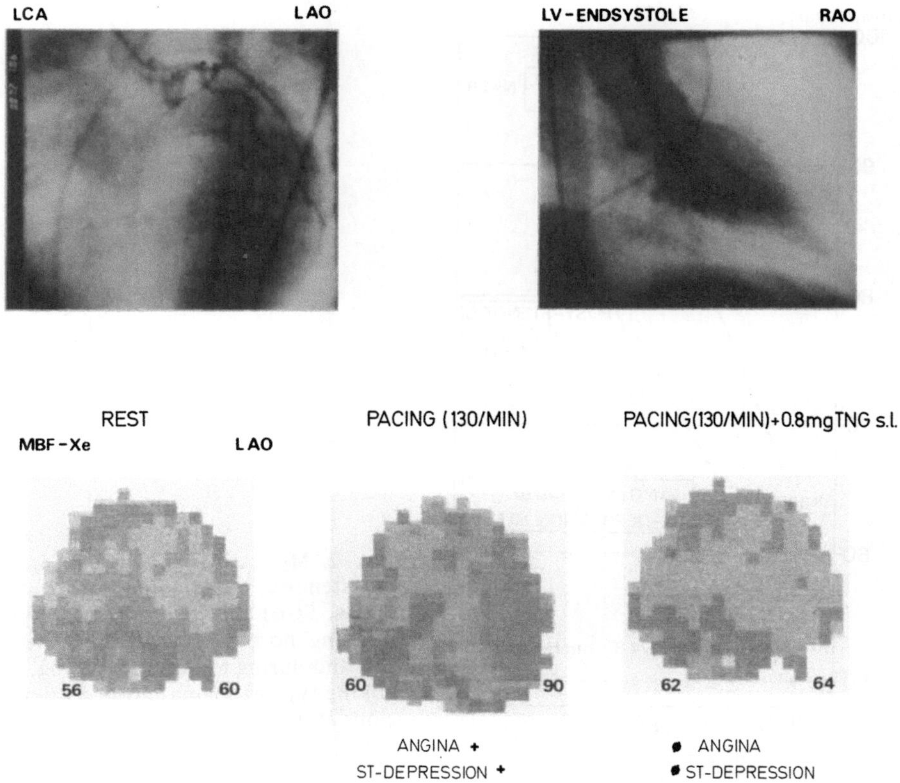

Fig. 1. Typical example of regional myocardial blood flow (ml/min per 100 g) in the normal and poststenotic area at rest, during atrial pacing and during pacing after administration of 0.8 mg nitroglycerin sublingually. *Above:* left coronary angiogram in the same *LAO* projection as the flow measurements were performed; it demonstrates a high degree obstruction of the *LAD*. *Right,* left ventricular angiogram in endsystole (*RAO* projection of 40°), demonstrating only minimal impairment of wall motion (hypokinesis) in the anterior region. *Below, from left to right,* flow image at rest, during rapid atrial pacing (*RAP*) up to angina and ST depressions of > 0.1 mV, and during RAP after administration of nitroglycerin. The flow image demonstrates the level of flow for each matrix point (*MP*), MPs in red indicating the highest flow values, the scale than decreasing to orange, yellow, green, and blue with the lowest flow values. *Note* that with pacing there was no increase in flow in the poststenotic area perfused by the LAD, whereas in the normal zone of the left circumflex branch, flow rose to 90 ml/min per 100 g (*red MPs*). After administration of nitroglycerin, flow was reduced especially in the normal zone, being now equal to the poststenotic zone (62 and 64 ml/min per 100 g myocardium, respectively), an expression of the marked reduction of oxygen demand (for details see text)

stenotic area for both groups (56.5 vs 56.3 ml/min per 100 g, respectively); however in the patients with coronary obstruction < 90%, RMBF increased to a significantly higher level of 83.5 ml/min per 100 g (+ 27 ml/min per 100 g (+ 48%)) than in the groups with obstructions > 90%, where it rose by 15.7 ml/min per 100 g (+ 27.8%),

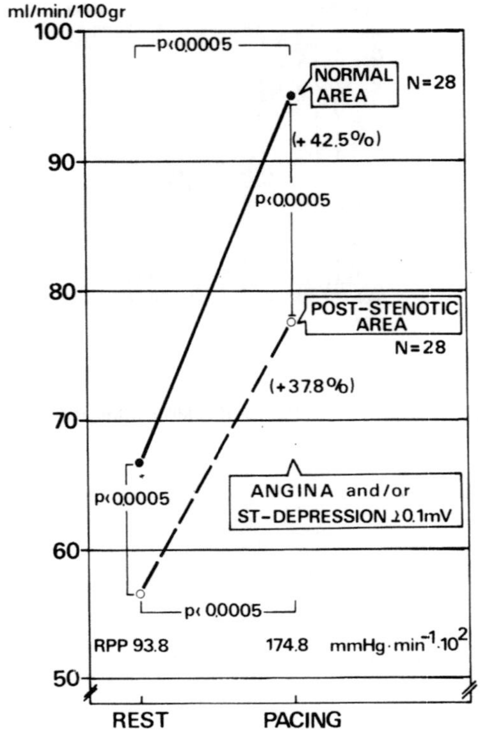

Fig. 2. Myocardial blood flow in the poststenotic (with stenoses > 90% and < 90%) (*broken line*) and corresponding normal zone (*heavy line*) at rest and during rapid atrial pacing, provoking typical angina and/or ST depressions ⩾ 0.1 mV

reaching 72 ml/min per 100 g. This difference in the maximum level of RMBF reached in both groups was highly significant ($P < 0.025$). It should be noted that in the normal area of these patients, no difference in RMBF was found either with regard to the resting stage (64.2 vs 69.1 ml/min per 100 g) or the level reached during RAP (93.5 and 96.5 ml/min per 100 g, respectively). Hence, in these 28 patients, RMBF during pacing-induced ischemia was significantly lower in patients with a higher degree of obstruction (> 90%) and/or collateral flow than in those with lower degrees of obstructions (⩽ 90%).

It is interesting to note that in three of the 28 patients, two with complete obstruction of the LAD and one with complete obstruction of the RCA, all with collateral filling only, transmural coronary flow actually decreased during atrial pacing by 2.1%, 7.5%, and 18.7% (Fig. 4); all three patients suffered from very severe angina during the study. Figure 5 demonstrates the behavior of RMBF in the four patients with the most severe angina during pacing in comparison to the five cases without angina or only mild chest discomfort, yet typical ST depressions. Heart rate and RPP were, with 143 vs 125 beats/min and 183 vs 158 mm Hg $\cdot$ $min^{-1} \cdot 10^{-2}$, considerably higher in the group without angina; the differences, however, were not significant.

It is interesting to note that, as mentioned above, in three of the four patients with the most severe angina, poststenotic regional myocardial blood flow actually decreased; due to the marked increase in RMBF in one case, the average remained unchanged from rest to rapid atrial pacing (67.4 vs 67.7 ml/min per 100 g, respectively). In patients without angina, poststenotic RMBF increased by 50% from 51 to 77 ml/min per

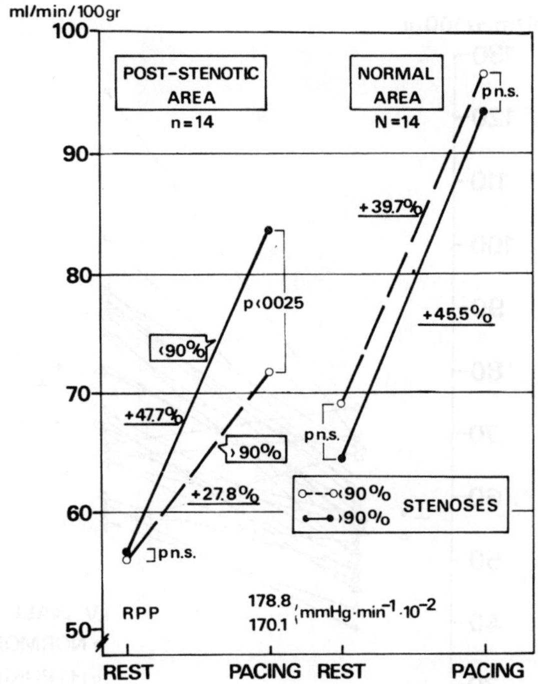

Fig. 3. Myocardial blood flow in the poststenotic areas (*left*) with stenosis ⩾ 90% and < 90% in the corresponding normal areas of the same patients (*right*) (for details see text)

100 g ($P < 0.01$); this, although at rest, was significantly lower in the latter group than in the patients developing severe angina (51.3 vs 67.4 ml/min per 100 g, $P < 0.025$).

Discussion

This study confirms in man the concept that during ischemia coronary blood flow is insufficient with regard to oxygen demand and delivery. In all patients studied here, who during rapid right atrial pacing suffered from typical angina pectoris or at least exhibited ST depressions > 0.1 mV, myocardial blood flow was significantly lower in the region perfused by a coronary artery with a high-grade obstruction (> 75%) than in the myocardial area perfused by a normal coronary artery. Furthermore, in three patients, all with severe angina, transmural poststenotic flow even decreased. These findings are therefore in good agreement with those published earlier by Schmidt [21], Maseri [15], and Cannon [2], all of whom also recorded regional myocardial blood flow during rapid atrial pacing, using gamma cameras and the precordial ^{133}xenon clearance technique. It is well known that the precordial xenon clearance technique used to register myocardial blood flow with the aid of gamma cameras has a number of disadvantages [11] asking for constraint regarding the interpretation of these data. The high affinity of xenon for adipose tissue, the lack of uniformity for the partition coef-

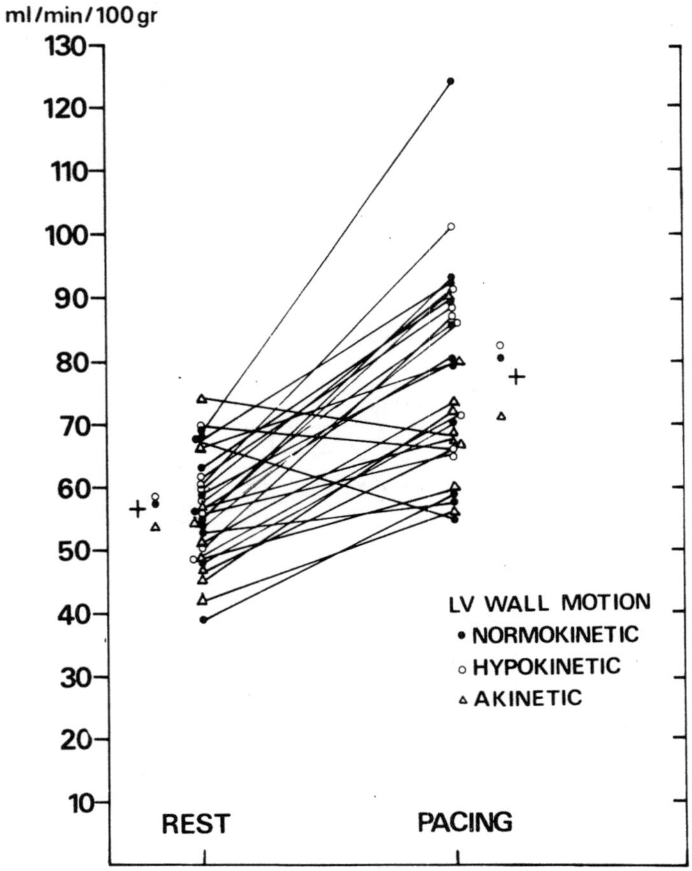

Fig. 4. Myocardial blood flow in the ischemic zone. This figure demonstrates individual results at rest and during rapid atrial pacing. Note that in three patients flow decreased, two of them having hypokinetic or normokinetic poststenotic wall motion at rest (for details see text)

ficient throughout the heart and the problems of geometry during rapid atrial pacing arising from the fast moving heart, are only a few of those constraints which could be mentioned. For these reasons, flow was only calculated for the center of large myocardial areas; overlapping border zones, where a considerable "smear effect" between normal and abnormal flow was expected, were excluded. A further disadvantage, of special importance for this study, lies in the fact that the gamma camera – although able to produce spatial separation – records transmural flow representing all layers of the myocardium. In addition to the inability to distinguish between epi- and endocardial flow, the xenon technique favors areas with rapid washout, slow washout curves from areas with low flow influencing those with rapid washout to only minor degree. Thus, if epicardial flow is high and endocardial flow unchanged or even mildly decreased, as demonstrated in animal studies during ischemia and in the presence of an elevated enddiastolic pressure [19], transmural flow will still increase. Only if endo-

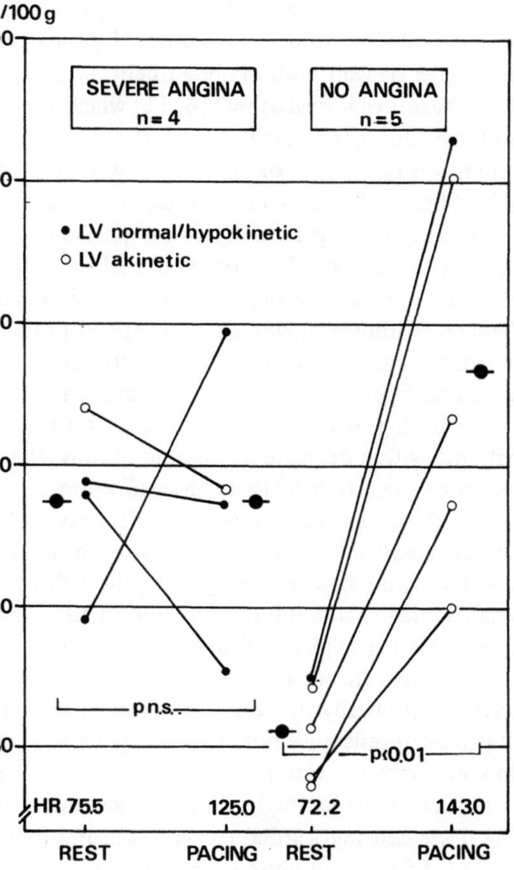

Fig. 5. RMBF in patients with severe angina during rapid atrial pacing (*left*) and in five patients without angina, yet typical ST depressions (*right*). Note that in three of the four patients with the most severe angina, flow decreased during rapid atrial pacing, whereas it uniformly increased in all patients without angina; furthermore, in four of the five patients without angina poststenotic wall motion was akinetic, i.e., small apical infarctions were present whereas three of the four with severe angina had a normal poststenotic wall motion or only mild hypokinesis

cardial flow and a large portion of flow in the middle layers of the myocardium decrease markedly, will transmural flow also decrease in spite of a mild increase in epicardial flow. Thus, the increase in transmural flow observed in 25 of the 28 patients does not exclude a decrease in flow in the endocardial zone during ischemia.

Furthermore, from angiographic [24, 25] as well as from radionuclide studies [1], it became evident that during exercise-induced ischemia, large portions of the poststenotic left ventricular wall segment are akinetic. Thus, impaired wall motion together with the resulting abnormal increase in left ventricular enddiastolic pressure, will further decrease myocardial blood flow in the poststenotic area. This was probably the case in the three patients with severe angina and decreased transmural flow.

Hence, during stress induced by rapid atrial pacing, the behavior of poststenotic flow is probably influenced not only by the degree of obstructions, but in addition by the degree of wall motion impairment, i.e., of ischemia. Nevertheless, this differs from the behavior observed at rest [4, 11] where flow was found to be dependent mainly on wall motion of the poststenotic region, i.e., oxygen demand and to a much lesser extent, on the degree of coronary obstruction. Patients with a typical old myocardial infarction in the ECG and corresponding akinetic areas in the left ventricular angiogram showed a significantly lower poststenotic myocardial blood flow at rest than those with normal left ventricular wall motion regardless of the degree of obstruction [11]. In contrast, during pacing-induced ischemia and markedly increased oxygen demand, coronary flow seems to depend primarily on the degree of the proximal obstruction. Patients with > 90% obstructions or occlusions of a coronary artery and collateral filling of the poststenotic area showed a significantly smaller increase in flow during pacing than those with coronary obstructions of ⩽ 90%. In addition, in all three patients with a decrease in transmural flow, the coronary arteries involved were totally occluded; yet, two of them showed normal poststenotic left ventricular wall motion at rest. This resulted in large ischemic areas during pacing. On the other hand, it was to be expected that in the presence of myocardial infarctions, i.e., akinetic areas due to scar tissue, no angina or only mild chest discomfort would result, corresponding to a small ischemic not infarcted region. This was the case in 4 of 5 of the 28 patients demonstrating typical ST depressions during pacing, yet no angina. Thus, it appears that the insufficient rise of coronary flow in the poststenotic area during rapid atrial pacing is primarily the result of the fixed high-grade proximal obstruction, the increase in proximal resistance not being compensated for even by maximal arteriolar dilatation; this indicates a severe reduction in coronary reserve. Nevertheless, it should be emphasized that ischemia might initiate a secondary mechanism of flow reduction based on the decreased myocardial oxygen consumption of the poststenotic wall segment, now excluded from contraction. Thus, the sustained lack of an adequate rise in poststenotic flow during rapid atrial pacing has to be explained both by anatomical and functional factors.

In spite of its limitations, the study confirms the present concept of ischemic heart disease in man by demonstrating that during increased hemodynamic activity, i.e., myocardial performance, ischemia is the result of the inability of regional flow to increase in accordance with oxygen demand. In this situation, the limitation is due to proximal coronary obstructions, mainly of a fixed, anatomical type. All further characteristics of the ischemic stage, especially the abnormal gradient of transmural flow, i.e., the decrease in endocardial flow, are also in agreement with the results of this study. Nevertheless, it should be remembered that stress induced ischemia is a complex situation accompanied by many secondary events [23], again influencing flow and wall motion.

Summary

Regional myocardial blood flow was studied at rest and during rapid atrial pacing in 28 patients with severe coronary artery disease (obstructions > 75%) using the precordial ^{133}xenon residue detection technique. During pacing averaging 142 beats/

min, flow increased significantly less in the poststenotic areas than in the normal zones ($P < 0.0005$); in the patients with severe angina and profound ST depression, transmural flow even decreased. The level of regional myocardial blood flow reached during atrial pacing was dependent on the degree of coronary obstruction: it was significantly lower in areas perfused by coronary arteries with obstruction > 90% or complete occlusions where coronary flow depended entirely on collaterals, than in those perfused by coronary arteries with obstructions of less than 90%. Thus, this study confirms in man the hypothesis derived from animal experiments, namely that there is a reduced poststenotic flow, i.e., insufficient oxygen delivery, during ischemia.

References

1 Borer JS, Bacharach SL, Green MV, Kent KM, Epstein SE, Johnson GS (1977) Real-time radionuclide cineangiography in the non-invasive evaluation of global and regional left ventricular function at rest and during exercise in patients with coronary artery disease. N Engl J Med 296:839

2 Cannon PJ, Weiss MB, Sciacca RR (1977) Myocardial blood flow in coronary artery disease: Studies at rest and during stress with inert gas washout techniques. Prog Cardiovasc Dis 20:95

3 Conti CR, Pitt B, Gundel WD, Friesinger GC, Ross RS (1970) Myocardial blood flow in pacing-induced angina. Circulation 42:815

4 Engel H-J, Lichtlen PR, Hundeshagen H (1977) Effects of coronary obstructions and segmental LV dysfunction on regional myocardial blood flow. Circulation 55/56:III–10

5 Gould KL (1980) Dynamic coronary stenosis. Am J Cardiol 45:286

6 Gould KL, Lipscomb K, Hamilton GW (1974) Physiologic basis for assessing critical coronary stenosis. Instantaneous flow response and regional distribution during coronary hyperemia as measures of coronary flow reserve. Am J Cardiol 33:87

7 Gould KL, Lipscomb K, Calvert C (1975) Compensatory changes of the distal coronary vascular bed during progressive coronary constriction. Cirulation 51:1085

8 Holmberg S, Varnauskas E (1971) Coronary circulation during pacing-induced tachycardia. Acta Med Scand 190:481

9 Holmberg S, Serzysko W, Varnauskas E (1971) Coronary circulation during heavy exercise in control subjects and patients with coronary heart disease. Acta Med Scand 190:465

10 Lichtlen PR (1977) Myocardial blood flow during exercise in patients with coronary artery disease. Herz 2:31

11 Lichtlen PR, Engel H-J (1979) Assessment of regional myocardial blood flow using the inert gas washout technique. Cardiovasc Radiol 2:203

12 Lipscomb K, Gould KL (1975) Mechanism of the effect of coronary artery stenosis on coronary flow in the dog. Am Heart J 80:60

13 Lichtlen P, Moccetti T, Halter J, Schönbeck M, Senning A (1972) Postoperative evaluation of myocardial blood flow in aorto-to coronary vein bypass using the Xenon-residue-detection technique. Circulation 46:445

14 Lichtlen PR, Engel H-J, Hundeshagen H (1978) Clinical application and results of the assessment of coronary blood flow by the regional precordial Xenon residue detection technique. Nucl Med 17:161

15 Maseri A, L'Abbate A, Pesola A, Michelassi C, Marzilli M, de Nes M (1977) Regional perfusion in patients with atherosclerotic coronary artery disease, at rest and during angina pectoris induced by tachycardia. Circulation 55:423

16 Nakamura M, Matsuguchi H, Mitsutake A, Kikuchi Y, Takeshita A, Nakagaki O, Kuroiwa A (1977) The effect of graded coronary stenosis on myocardial blood flow and left ventricular wall motion. Basic Res Cardiol 72:479
17 Rafflenbeul W, Lichtlen PR (1979) Intravital morphometrie. In: Lichten PR (ed) Koronarangiographie. Straube, Erlangen, p 325
18 Rafflenbaul W, Smith LR, Rogers WJ, Mantle JA, Rackley JE, Russell RO, Freudenberg H, Lichtlen P (1980) Koronarmorphologie bei Patienten mit unstabiler Angina pectoris. Herz 5:25
19 Schaper W (1979) Residual perfusion of actuely ischemic heart muscle. In: Schaper W (ed) The pathophysiology of myocardial perfusion. Elsevier/North Holland, Amsterdam, p 345
20 Schaper W, Wüsten B, Flameng W, Scholtholt J, Winkler B, Pasky St (1975) Local dilatory reserve in chronic experimental coronary occlusions without infarction. Quantitation of collateral development. Basic Res Cardiol 70:159
21 Schmidt DH, Weiss MB, Casarella WJ, Fowler DL, Sciacca RR, Cannon PJ (1976) Regional myocardial perfusion during atrial pacing in patients with coronary artery disease. Circulation 53:807
22 Schwarz F (1979) Correlation between the degree of coronary artery obstruction and myocardial dysfunction. In: Schaper W (ed) The pathophysiology of myocardial perfusion. Elsevier/North Holland Biomedical Press, Amsterdam, p 305
23 Selwyn AP, Kim F, Clay T (1979) The effect of acute regional myocardial ischemia on the angiographic anatomy of coronary arteries. Circulation 60:1335
24 Sharma B, Goodwin JF, Raphael MJ, Steiner RE, Rainbow RG, Taylor SH (1976) Left ventricular angiography on exercise. A new method of assessing left ventricular function in ischemic heart disease. Br Heart J 38:59
25 Sigwart U, Schmidt H, Bonzel T, Mertens HM, Gleichmann U (1975) Biplane cineangiographic evaluation of left ventricular contraction in ischemic heart disease at rest and during bicycle exercise. Circulation 51/52:II–37
26 Simon R, Amende I, Lichtlen PR (1979) Das linksventrikuläre Angiogramm. In: Lichtlen PR (ed) Koronarangiographie. Straube, Erlangen, p 249

Part III
ECG and Coronarography

Comparison of Exercise ECG and Coronary Angiography

H. Roskamm and L. Samek

Introduction

Exercise tests and coronary arteriography reflect two different aspects of coronary heart disease: functional and anatomic. Moreover, the relationships between these two methods depend on the selection of patients; prevalence of coronary artery disease plays an important role [1].

The following questions will be discussed in this article:

1. What is the correlation between the results of exercise tests and the results of coronary arteriography in patients *without* previous myocardial infarction?
2. Is there a correlation between exercise parameters and the severity of coronary artery disease?
3. Can exercise tests predict involvement of a second or third vessel in patients *with* previous myocardial infarction?
4. What were the preoperative results of exercise tests in patients with left main stem stenosis who were operated on?
5. What is the correlation between the results of exercise tests and the degree of revascularization in patients after aortocoronary bypass surgery?

Methods

Exercise tests were performed in the supine position on a bicycle ergometer, starting at 25 or 50 W, increasing every 6 min by 25 or 50 W without interruption, until severe angina pectoris, life-threatening arrhythmias, severe fatigue, or dyspnea occurred (symptom-limited test). The test was judged as negative if at least 80% of the age-predicted maximal heart rate (220 minus age in years) was reached without symptoms and signs.

Coronary arteriography was performed by the Sones or Judkins technique in several projections including caudocranial. The results of the exercise tests were compared with the results of coronary arteriography.

Results

Study I: Patients Without Transmural Myocardial Infarction with Proven or Suspected Angina Pectoris in Their History [2]

In 311 patients (269 men and 42 women, 20–65 years old) without transmural myocardial infarction, the correlations between exercise test and coronary arteriography were as follows:

Of the patients with angina pectoris and ST segment depression (> 0.1 mV) during exercise (n = 108), 86.1% showed a > 50% stenosis of at least one vessel (Fig. 1). The number of men having a > 50% stenosis was significantly higher than the number of women (91.3% vs 56.2%). If only one ischemia indicator was positive, only 30% and 37%, respectively, of the patients showed a significant stenosis. In patients having neither angina pectoris nor ST segment depression up to 80% of the age-dependent heart rate limit, the incidence of a significant stenosis was still 12.4%, but 11 of 13 patients had one-vessel disease and had already suffered an intramural infarction. There was no patient with three-vessel disease in this group. The number of positive coronary angiograms, especially of two- and three-vessel disease, increased with the degree of ST segment depression and the reduction of exercise tolerance. In patients with an exercise tolerance of 100 W or more, three-vessel disease was very rare (Fig. 2).

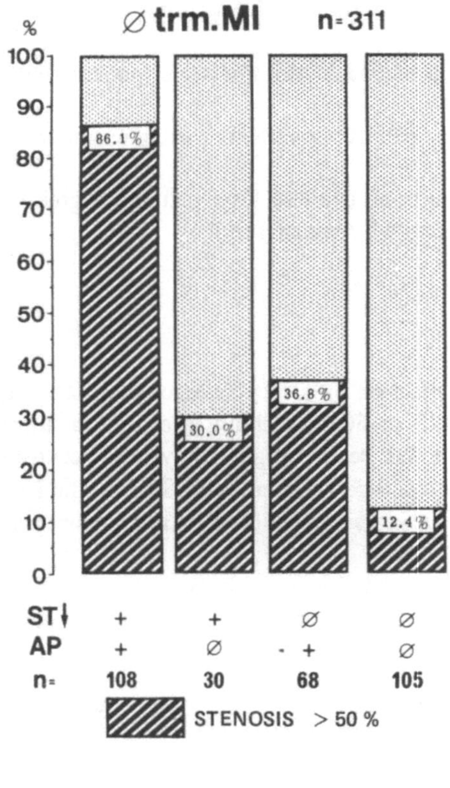

Fig. 1. Incidence of a > 50% stenosis of at least one coronary artery in relation to ST segment depression (ST ↓) and angina pectoris (*AP*) during exercise in 311 patients without transmural myocardial infarction (*trm. MI*)

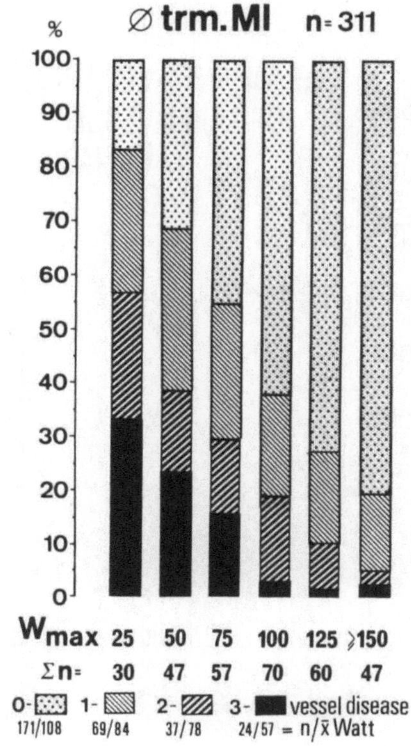

Fig. 2. Frequency of one-, two-, or three-vessel disease (stenosis > 50%) in relation to maximum exercise tolerance in watts in the supine position. Patient material as in Fig. 1. *trm. MI*, transmural myocardial infarction

Study II: Postinfarction Patients With or Without Angina Pectoris More Than 8 Weeks After the Acute Event [3]

Two hundred and sixty one postinfarction patients (mean age 46 years, range 29–62 years) were investigated in order to see whether involvement of a second and third vessel could be predicted on the basis of angina pectoris and/or ST segment depression during exercise. The main findings were as follows.

Severe lesions (> 75%) of a second or third vessel were found in 61.7% of patients with inferior myocardial infarction who developed angina pectoris and ST segment depression in the anterior leads during exercise (Fig. 3). In patients with neither angina pectoris nor ST segment depression during exercise, only 3.4% had multivessel disease. If only one ischemia indicator was positive, multivessel disease was present in 18.6% and 9.1%, respectively. In patients with anteroseptal infarction the correlations were not so clear cut. But also in this group patients with neither angina pectoris nor ST segment depression during exercise again very seldom had multivessel disease.

Study III: Patients with Left Main Stem Disease Who Were Surgically Treated

In 133 patients with left main stem stenosis of > 50% who were operated on, the mean age was 52.2 years (range 30–70 years, 96.2% being men). Coronary arteriographic

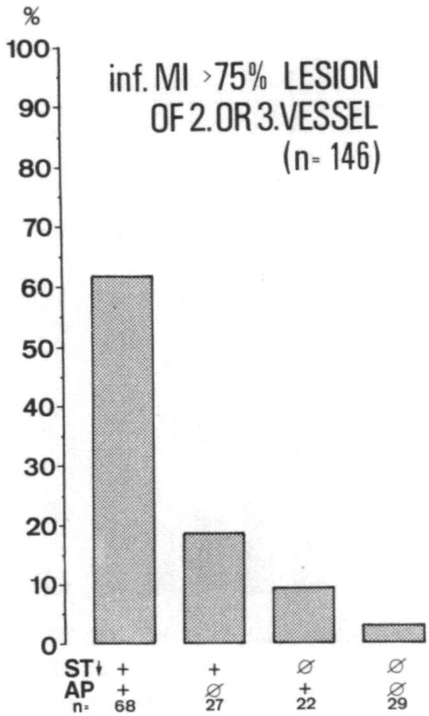

Fig. 3. Incidence of multivessel disease (> 75% stenosis) in patients at least 8 weeks after a transmural myocardial infarction (*inf. MI*) in relation to ST segment depression and angina pectoris during exercise

findings of this group are given in Table 1. Preoperative occurrence of angina pectoris and ST segment depression during maximal exercise and angina pectoris-free exercise tolerance are shown in Fig. 4. Patients having angina pectoris during exercise numbered 117. The majority of patients had an angina-free exercise tolerance below 50 W. An ST segment depression of 0.2 mV–0.5 mV and more was also present in the majority of patients. Thus, the majority shows very pronounced signs and symptoms of ischemia during exercise. But 16 patients had a rather high angina pectoris-free exercise tolerance of 75 W or more. Also, 31 patients had no ST segment depression or an ST segment depression of below 0.2 mV. Patients having no angina pectoris during exercise numbered 16. The combination, however, of high exercise tolerance and only slight ST segment depression during exercise is rare. Only five patients (4%) could exercise at 75 W or more with only slight ST segment depression of below 0.2 mV. Thus, only moderately limited exercise tolerance in patients with left main stem stenosis is rare, but it is possible.

Study IV: Coronary Heart Disease Patients After Aortocoronary Bypass Surgery

In 825 patients (mean age 51.5 years, range 24–71 years) in whom aortocoronary bypass surgery had been performed, the correlation between degree of revascularization (Table 2) and functional improvement after the operation was analyzed.

Table 1. Involvement of the different vessels (left anterior descending artery (LAD), left circumflex artery (LCx), and right coronary artery (RCA)) in 133 patients with a > 50% stenosis of the left main stem who were operated on. In only 7.5% of the patients was there a stenosis of only the left main stem. 2-VD and 3-VD, two- and three-vessel disease, respectively

Vessels with > 50% stenosis, n = 133					
LMCA	LAD	LCx	RCA		
+	●	●	●	7.5%	
+	+	●	●	5.3%	2-VD 22.6%
+	●	+	●	2.3%	
+	+	+	●	7.5%	
+	●	●	+	6.0%	
+	●	+	+	4.5%	3-VD 77.4%
+	+	●	+	14.3%	
+	+	+	+	52.6%	

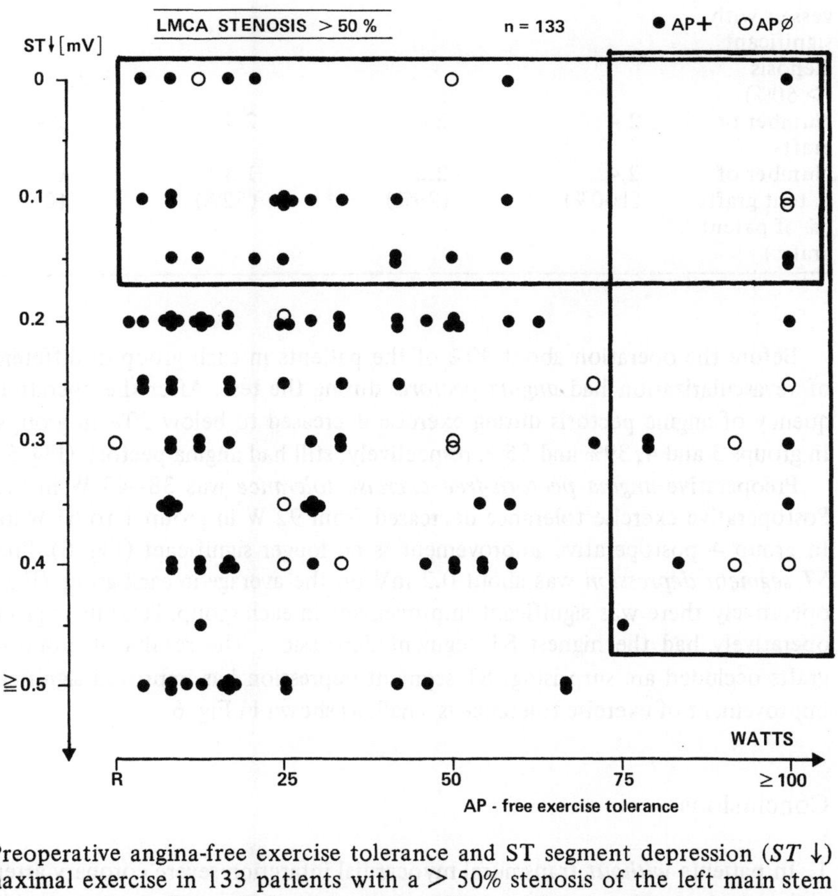

Fig. 4. Preoperative angina-free exercise tolerance and ST segment depression (*ST* ↓) during maximal exercise in 133 patients with a > 50% stenosis of the left main stem who were operated on. *Open circles* represent patients without angina pectoris during exercise

Table 2. Degree of revascularization and graft patency in 825 patients after aortocoronary bypass surgery. In the majority of patients postoperative angiography was performed about 1 year after the operation. In 74 patients a pre- and postoperative exercise test was not available, mainly because of severe angina pectoris at rest preoperatively which did not allow an exercise test

Degree of revascularization and graft patency (825 patients, 51.1 years, 777 men, 48 women, 2.6 grafts/patient)

Degree	1 (n = 336)	2 (n = 331)	3 (n = 123)	4 (n = 35)
Revascular.	Complete	Sufficient	Insufficient	Unsuccessful
Definition	All grafts to vessels with significant stenosis (> 50%) pat.	Grafts to most import. vessels (especially LAD patent)	Grafts to most import. vessels occluded, but at least one graft patent	All grafts occluded
Number of vessels with significant stenosis (> 50%)	2.3	2.7	2.7	2.1
Number of grafts	2.4	2.8	2.9	2.4
Number of patent grafts (% of patent grafts)	2.4 (100%)	2.2 (79%)	1.5 (52%)	0 (0%)

Before the operation about 90% of the patients in each group of different degrees of revascularization had *angina pectoris* during the test. After the operation the frequency of angina pectoris during exercise decreased to below 20% in groups 1 and 2. In groups 3 and 4, 39% and 55%, respectively, still had angina pectoris (Fig. 5).

Preoperative *angina pectoris-free exercise tolerance* was 38–43 W in each group. Postoperative exercise tolerance decreased from 92 W in group 1 to 61 W in group 4. In group 4 postoperative improvement is no longer significant (Fig. 6). Preoperative *ST segment depression* was about 0.2 mV on the average in each group (Fig. 7). Postoperatively there was significant improvement in each group. Patients in group 3 postoperatively had the highest ST segment depression. The results of group 4 with all grafts occluded are surprising: ST segment depression has improved significantly, but improvement of exercise tolerance is small, as shown in Fig. 6.

Conclusions

1. In patients *without* transmural myocardial infarction severe coronary artery disease is rare

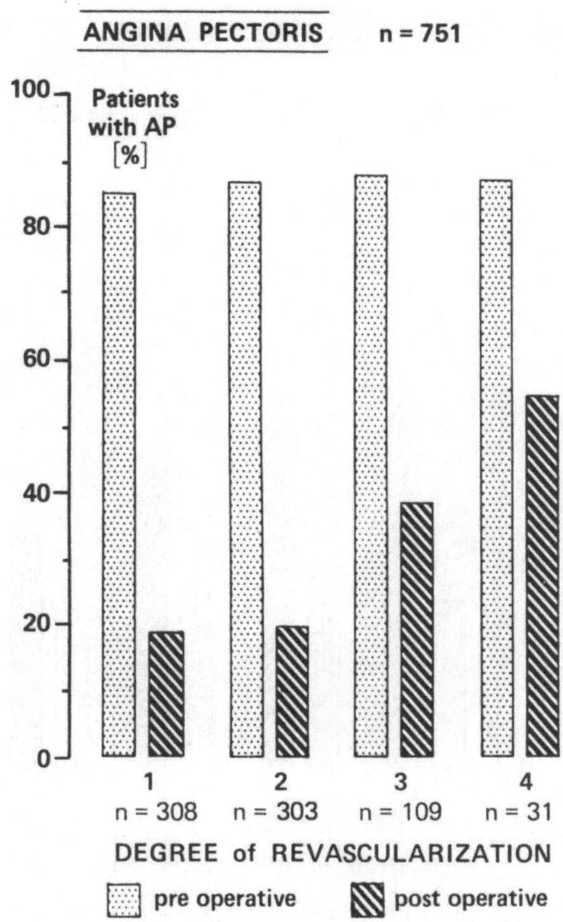

Fig. 5. Pre- and postoperative incidence of angina pectoris (*AP*) in 751 patients in whom aortocoronary bypass surgery was performed in relation to degree of revascularization (for definition see Table 2)

(a) in patients having neither angina pectoris nor ST segment depression during maximal exercise;
(b) in patients having only angina pectoris or ST segment depression during maximal exercise; and
(c) in patients achieving high levels of exercise.

2. In patients *with* transmural myocardial infarction critical stenosis of second or third vessel is rare if neither angina pectoris nor ST segment depression occurs during maximal exercise testing.
3. Patients with transmural inferior infarction who, 8 weeks following the infarction, develop angina pectoris and ST segment depression during exercise, have a high incidence of critical stenosis in a second or third vessel.

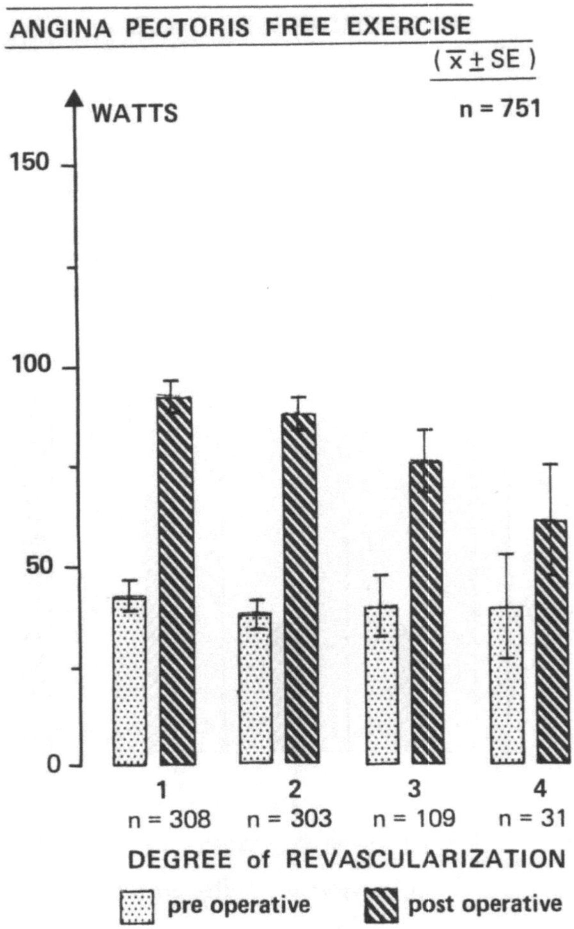

Fig. 6. Pre- and postoperative angina pectoris-free exercise tolerance in 751 patients in whom aortocoronary bypass surgery was performed in relation to degree of revascularization. Postoperative improvement in group 4 with all grafts occluded is not significant (for definition see Table 2)

4. Patients with left main stem disease usually show pronounced signs and symptoms of ischemia during exercise. Patients with a rather high exercise tolerance and only slight ST segment depression are rare but they exist.
5. In patients in whom aortocoronary bypass surgery was performed, postoperative functional improvement is different in groups of different degrees of revascularization, but relationships are not very close. In particular, some patients with all grafts occluded show an unexpected improvement after the operation.

These correlations between the results of the exercise test and the results of coronary arteriography may help to make the indications for coronary arteriography more precise.

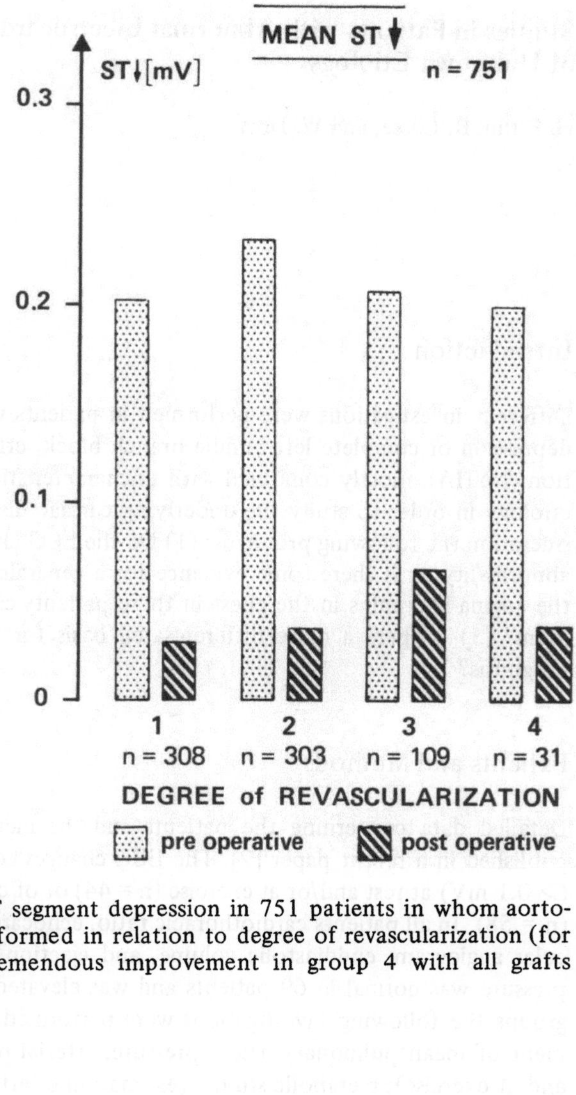

Fig. 7. Pre- and postoperative ST segment depression in 751 patients in whom aortocoronary bypass surgery was performed in relation to degree of revascularization (for definition see Table 2). The tremendous improvement in group 4 with all grafts occluded is surprising

References

1 Katz MA (1974) A probability graph describing the predictive value of a highly sensitive diagnostic test. N Engl J Med 291:1115

2 Roskamm H, Samek L, Zweigle K, Stürzenhofecker P, Petersen J, Rentrop P, Prokoph J (1977) Die Beziehungen zwischen den Befunden der Koronarangiographie und des Belastungs-EKG bei Patienten ohne transmuralen Myokardinfarkt. Z Kardiol 66:273

3 Samek L, Roskamm H, Rentrop P, Kaiser P, Stürzenhofecker P, Schober B, Görnandt L, Velden R (1975) Belastungsprüfungen und Koronarangiogramm im chronischen Infarktstadium. Z Kardiol 64:809

Studies in Patients with Abnormal Electrocardiogram of Unknown Etiology

H. Kuhn, B. Lösse, and W. Hort

Introduction

Different investigations were performed in patients with abnormal ECG (ST segment depression or complete left bundle branch block, criteria of New York Heart Association (NYHA), mostly combined with uncharacteristic pains in the chest) of unknown etiology in order to study the underlying cardiac disorder. The studies took into consideration the following problems: (1) Do the ECG changes represent only an electrical abnormality or is there some evidence for a generalized myocardial disorder? (2) Are the angina-like pains in the chest in these patients caused by ischemia of the myocardium? (3) Is there a more differentiated basis for follow-up studies to evaluate the prognosis?

Patients and Methods

Detailed data concerning the patients and the methods applied in this study were published in a recent paper [2]. The ECG changes consisted of ST segment depression (> 0.1 mV) at rest and/or at exercise (n = 44) or of complete left bundle branch block (n = 58). In all patients cardiothoracic ratio, echocardiogram, coronary and left ventricular angiogram, enddiastolic volume, and ejection fraction were normal. The aortic pressure was normal in 69 patients and was elevated in 33 patients. In different subgroups the following investigations were performed: hemodynamic studies (measurement of mean pulmonary artery pressure, arterial pressure, and cardiac index at rest and at exercise); metabolic studies (estimation of arteriocoronary venous difference of lactate, free fatty acids (FFA), glucose, and oxygen at rest and at high frequent atrial pacing); studies with radioactive isotopes (thallium-201 myocardial imaging and measurement of minimal cardiac transit times (indium-113) at rest and at exercise); and morphological studies (right ventricular endomyocardial catheter biopsy and light and electron microscopy).

Results

The results were reported and discussed in recent papers [1, 2, 3]. The rates of abnormal findings are summarized in Table 1. Data from two patients with ST segment depression of unknown etiology are shown in Fig. 1.

Table 1. Rate of abnormal findings in patients with abnormal ECG of unknown cause (normal echo- and coronary angiogram and normal ventriculogram)

Investigation	Rate of abnormal findings Total	n	LBBB	n	ST ↓	n
MPAP at exercise	53%	(50/95)	57%	(29/51)	48%	(21/44)
Extraction of lactate	47%	(24/51)	56%	(14/25)	39%	(10/26)
Scintigram	29%	(6/21)	100%	(4/4)	90%	(28/31)
McTT	29%	(6/21)	29%	(6/21)	–	–
Biopsy	83%	(45/54)	81%	(22/27)	85%	(23/27)

Abbreviations: MPAP, mean pulmonary artery pressure; *McTT*, minimal cardiac transit times; *LBBB*, patients with left bundle branch block; *ST* ↓, patients with ST segment depression at rest and/or at exercise

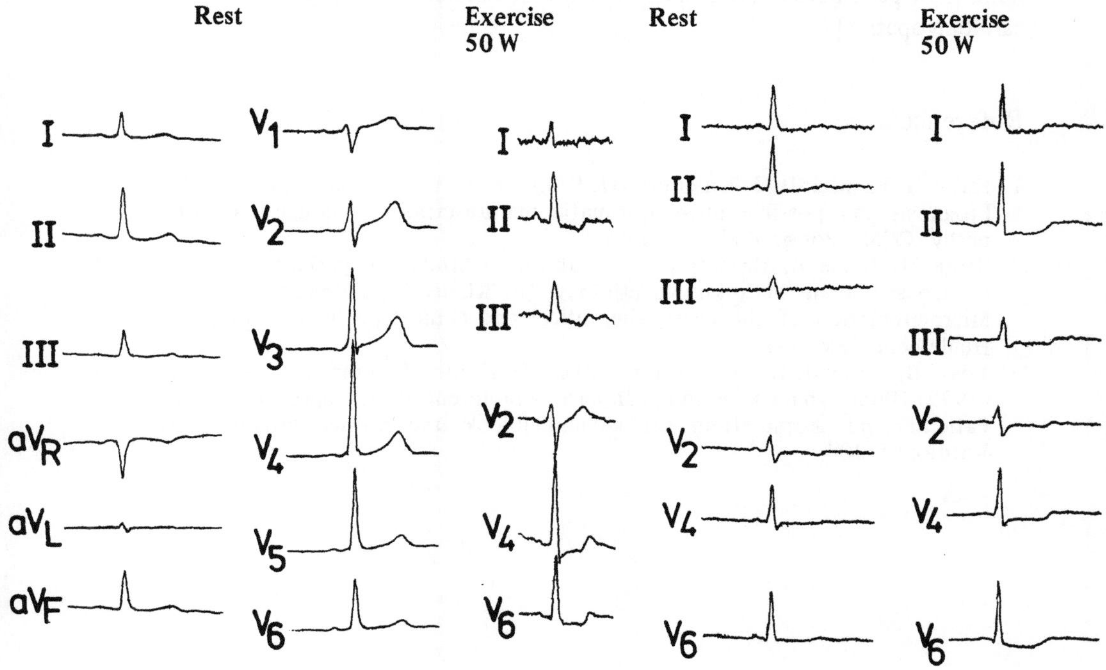

Fig. 1. Abnormal ST segment depression at exercise of unknown etiology in 42-year-old man (*left*) and a 53-year-old women (*right*). Arterial blood pressure, coronary angiogram, ventriculogram, and one- and two-dimensional echocardiograms were normal. The mean pulmonary artery pressure at exercise was abnormally elevated in the 42-year-old man, indicating impaired left ventricular function at exercise. In both patients a production of lactate was observed at high frequent atrial pacing. The scintigram showed perfusion defects at rest and at exercise, indicating coronary artery disease, and the endomyocardial catheter biopsy revealed abnormal findings in both patients consisting of interstitial fibrosis, hypertrophied muscle cells, and degenerative changes detectable electron microscopically

Conclusions

It is concluded that in a high rate of patients with abnormal ECG of unknown etiology, mostly combined with uncharacteristic chest pain, in spite of angiographically normal coronary arteries and normal echocardiogram and ventriculogram, a generalized myocardial disorder and ischemia or hypoxia of heart muscle at exercise seem to be present. Latent impairment of left ventricular function can also be found. Furthermore, the results do not support the posssibility that the myocardial disorder of these patients is caused by small-vessel disease; however, they also do not exclude this possibility. Finally, the data provide a more differentiated basis (absence or presence and degree of abnormal lactate extraction, of thallium-201 perfusion defects, of morphological abnormalities, and of abnormal elevation of mean pulmonary artery pressure with and without abnormal prolongation of minimal cardiac transit times) for follow-up studies to evaluate the prognoses of those patients, which today remain unclear. Only in patients with left bundle branch block is there different evidence that at least in a small number of patients the left bundle branch block indicates an early stage of congestive cardiomyopathy [1].

References

1 Kuhn H, Breithardt G, Knieriem HJ, Köhler E, Lösse B, Seipel L, Loogen F (1978) Prognosis and possible presymptomatic manifestations of congestive cardiomyopathy (CCM). Postgrad Med J 54:451

2 Kuhn H, Lösse B, Hort W (to be published) Studies in patients with abnormal electrocardiogram of unknown etiology. In: Kübler W, Tillmans H, Zebe H (eds) Microcirculation of the heart, theoretical and clinical problems. Springer, Berlin Heidelberg New York

3 Lösse B, Kuhn H, Krönert H, Rafflenbeul D, Köhler E, Schicha H, Feinendegen LE (1979) Hämodynamische und radiokardiographische Belastungsuntersuchungen bei Patienten mit komplettem Linksschenkelblock und normal großem Herzen. Z Kardiol 68:304

Ventricular Arrhythmias and Angiographic Findings

K.P. Bethge and P.R. Lichtlen

Problem

Why this unusual correlation? Ventricular extrasystoles (VES) have been shown to be of prognostic significance in patients with coronary artery disease (CAD) [8, 9, 11, 14, 15, 20, 21]. On the other hand coronary and left ventricular angiography has proved to be the technique with the highest reliability in predicting survival of coronary patients [4, 5, 6, 10, 13, 17, 22]. In order to get more detailed profiles of patients at increased risk of sudden death it seemed promising to correlate rhythm analysis with angiographic findings [1, 2, 3, 7].

Patients

We examined 223 patients – 198 males and 25 females – undergoing coronary and left ventricular angiography using either the Sones or the Judkins technique. One hundred and sixty seven consecutive patients – according to daily capacities of the tape recorders – showed CAD; 158 of them were male (mean age 50.2; range 36–65) and nine female (mean age 53.3; range 41–65). Additionally, 56 patients with normal coronary arteries, with normal left ventricular wall motion, and normal hemodynamic findings were included in this study needing a significantly longer inclusion period in comparison to the aforementioned coronary group. This "normal" control group consisted of 40 males (mean age 46.8; range 27–66) and 16 females (mean age 50.9; range 36–64).

Rhythm Analysis

Since long-term ECG monitoring has become the superior method in detecting cardiac arrhythmias, ECGs were stored on tapes over periods of 24 h during the days following cardiac catheterization using a light-weight (450 g) portable tape recorder (Oxford Electronic Instruments). Every medication was withdrawn at least 2 days before with the exception of digitalis in patients with congestive heart failure (classes III and IV NYHA) and with the exception of nitrates in patients with severe angina.

High-speed tape analysis was performed at 60 times the real time with the support of the Neilson arrhythmia computer [16] using a modified Pathfinder RME (Reynolds Medical Electronics, London), essentially completed by means of a CBS module (Emetron GmbH, Munich). This system was recently described in detail [18].

Although the excellent reliability of the Neilson arrhythmia computer in detecting ectopic activity (both sensitivity and specificity > 90%) is well known [12, 19], the more complex arrhythmias (couplets, salvos, ventricular tachycardia, and RR intervals > 200 ms) were validated by visual analysis from recording (25 mm/s) of each such episode.

Results

Incidence of Ventricular Dysrhythmias

To characterize the incidence of ventricular dysrhythmias for a storage period of 24 h we use a logarithmic scale given in Fig. 1a. The second scale below refers to the hourly incidence of VES. This is of theoretical interest only because of the remarkable spontaneous variability of VES within 24 h. As the distribution clearly demonstrates, more than 30% of the patients show a high incidence of VES (> 240 VES/24 h).

Since several reports in the literature have suggested that complex forms of VES coincide with poor prognosis [11, 14, 15, 20, 21] the incidence of complex arrhythmias is of particular interest. For this reason we use a modified Lown classification of VES [14] given in Fig. 2a and b. Interestingly, all the dysrhythmias in Fig. 2 were recorded from a 54-year-old male patient 4 weeks after anterior myocardial infarction showing a severe (> 75%) proximal obstruction of the left anterior descending branch.

Using this classification of VES, 51% of the entire group shows no or only a moderate incidence of VES (grades 0 and I) in contrast to 25% being in classes IV and V (Fig. 1b). So nearly one-third of the study group show a high incidence as well as complex forms of ventricular dysrhythmias.

VES in "Normal" Subjects and Coronary Patients

The distribution of VES in Fig. 1a changes significantly with the separation into a "normal" control group and patients with documented CAD (Fig. 3a). Of the "normal" subjects 73% (41/56) show VES sporadically (0–24 VES/24 h). In contrast, this low incidence of ectopic activity is seen in only 34% of the coronary patients (57/167), the majority of whom have an increased ectopic activity. As statistical analysis confirms, coronary patients produce significantly more ectopic activity than "normal" controls ($P < 0.0005$).

An analogous finding can be demonstrated according to maximal grading of VES (Fig. 3b). Of the "normal" subjects, 80% (45 patients) show no or only a moderate incidence of VES (grades 0 and I) in contrast to only 41% (69) of coronary patients. Spontaneous repetitive ectopic activity (black bars) is observed in 7% (four patients) of the "normals" in comparison to 31% (51) of the coronary patients. So again, between "normal" subjects and patients with CAD there is a highly significant difference of VES according to Lown's grading of ectopic activity ($P < 0.0005$). The underlying disease seems to be a determining factor in the genesis of ventricular arrhythmias.

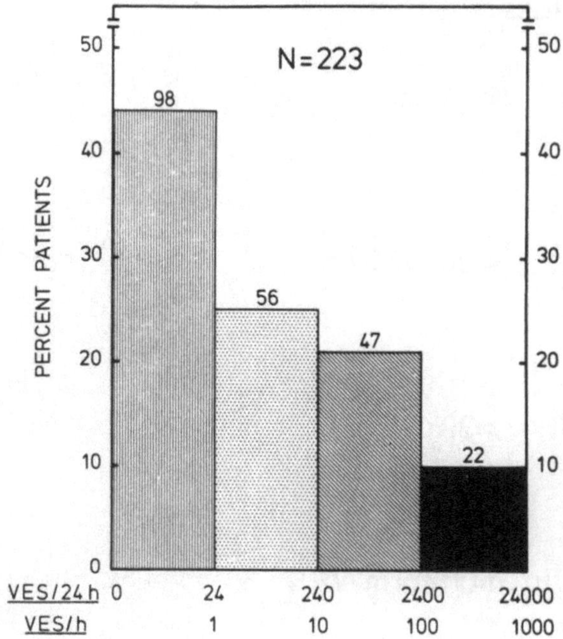

Fig. 1. a Incidence of ventricular extrasystoles (*VES*) in patients undergoing coronary angiography. The figures above the bars indicate number of patients whereas the height of the bars reflect percentage of the entire group discussed. Further details see text

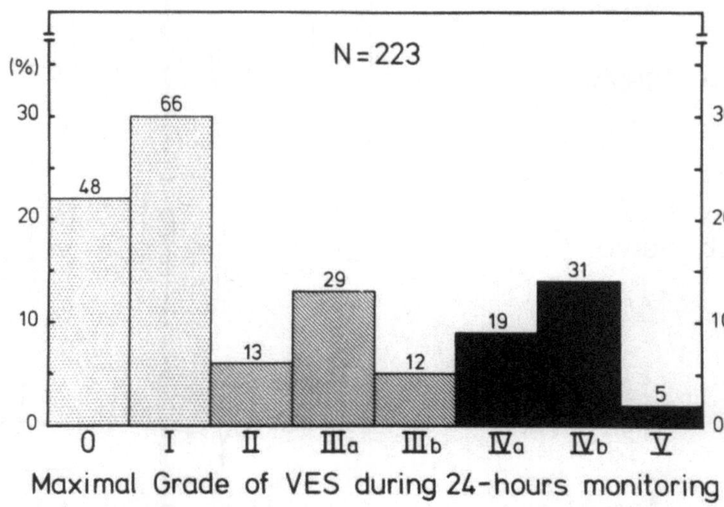

Fig. 1. b Maximal grading of *VES* in patients undergoing coronary angiography

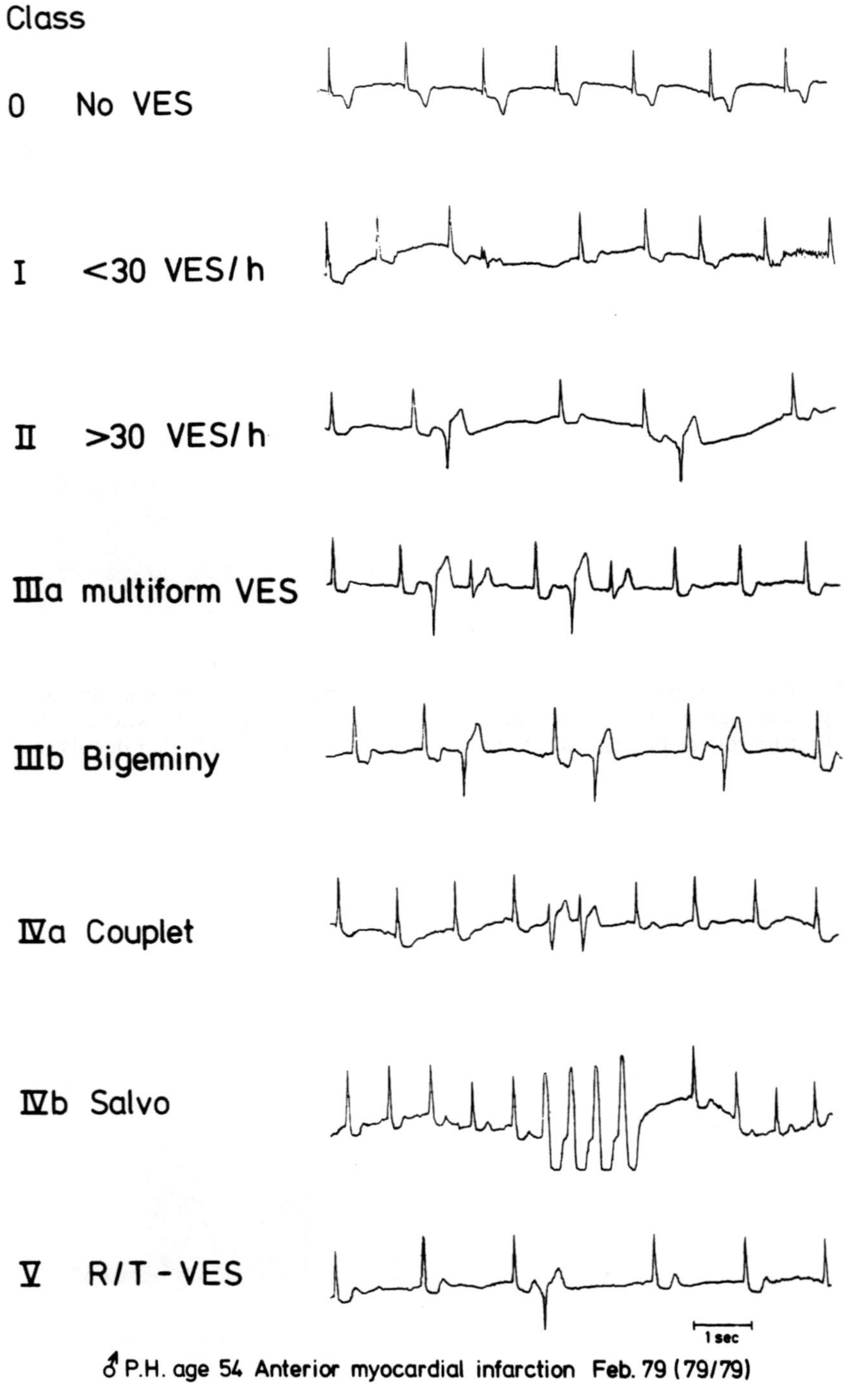

Fig. 2a, b. Modified Lown classification of *VES*; the modification refers to the introduction of bigeminal rhythm (class IIIb). Interestingly, all these ventricular dysrhythmias were seen in a 54-year-old male patient 4 weeks after anterior myocardial infarction

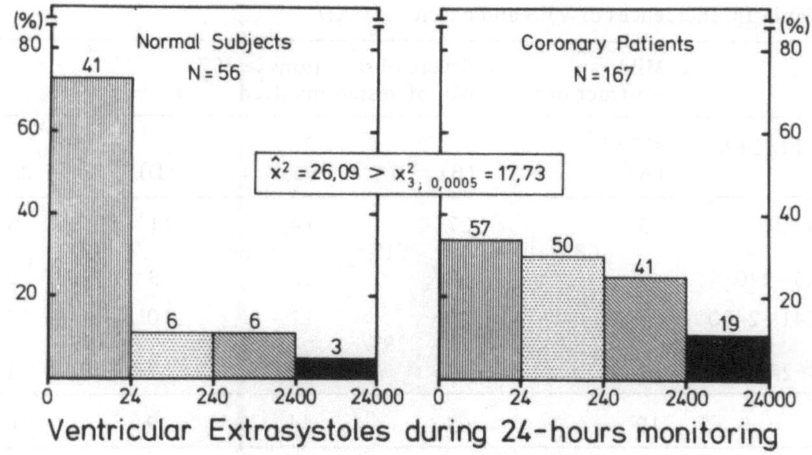

Fig. 3. a Incidence of *VES* in "normal" subjects and coronary patients

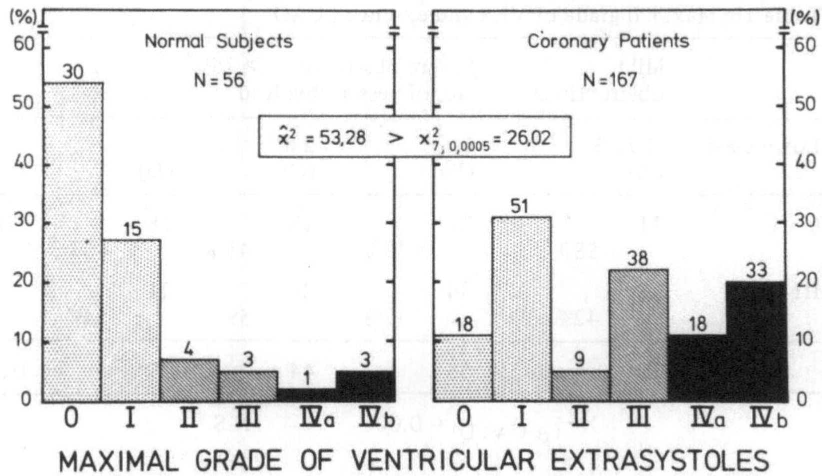

Fig. 3. b Maximal grading of *VES* in "normal" subjects and coronary patients

Ectopic Activity in Relation to the Extent of CAD

Focusing on the group of coronary patients we analyzed the incidence of VES in relation to the angiographic extent of CAD. As shown in Table 1a there is a clear trend toward a rising number of VES with an increasing number of vessels involved ($P < 0.06$). This relationship is even more convincing after excluding the group with only mild obstructions (< 75%) of coronary artery ($P < 0.05$). Of patients with three-vessel disease 49% exhibit high ectopic activity (> 240 VES/24 h) in comparison to 34% with two-vessel disease and only 29% of patients with one-vessel disease.

Table 1a. Incidences of VES and extent of CAD

	Mild. obstructions		Severe obstructions > 75% No. of vessels involved							
VES/24 h	< 75% (A)		1 (B)		2 (C)		3 (D)		Σ	
0–24	5		27		14		11		57	
		63%		71%		66%		51%		64%
25–240	7		19		15		9		50	
241–2400	5		15		11		10		41	
		37%		29%		34%		49%		36%
> 2400	2		4		4		9		19	
Σ	19		65		44		39		167	

X^2 (A-C vs D) = 3.62 P < 0.06

Table 1b. Maximal grade of VES and extent of CAD

	Mild obstructions		Severe obstructions > 75% No. of vessels involved							
Lown class	< 75% (A)		1 (B)		2 (C)		3 (D)		Σ	
0–II	11		31		18		18		78	
		58%		48%		41%		46%		47%
III–V	8		34		26		21		89	
		42%		52%		59%		54%		53%
Σ	19		65		44		39		167	

X^2 (A-C vs D) = 0.006 N.S.

Since VES Lown grades III–V may have prognostic implications we divided coronary patients into two major groups (Table 1b). No relationship can be demonstrated between the number of involved vessels and these major groups. There are no significant differences between the eight groups. This is probably due to the fact that 50% (84) of coronary patients show multiform VES. Such frequent occurrence of a criterion does not allow sensitive discrimination.

Ectopic Activity in Relation to Left Ventricular Wall Motion

In contrast to the degree of involvement of coronary arteries, there is a highly significant correlation between regional left ventricular wall motion abnormalities and the incidence of VES (Fig. 4a). Of Coronary patients with akinetic wall motion, 46%

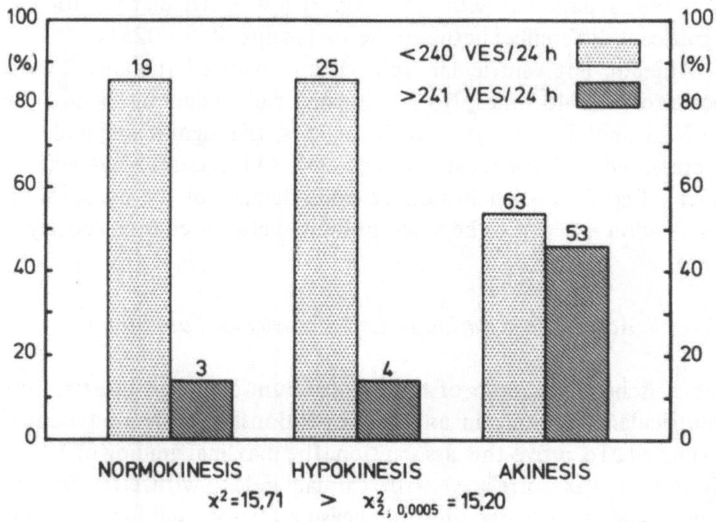

Fig. 4. a Incidence of *VES* in relation to left ventricular wall motion

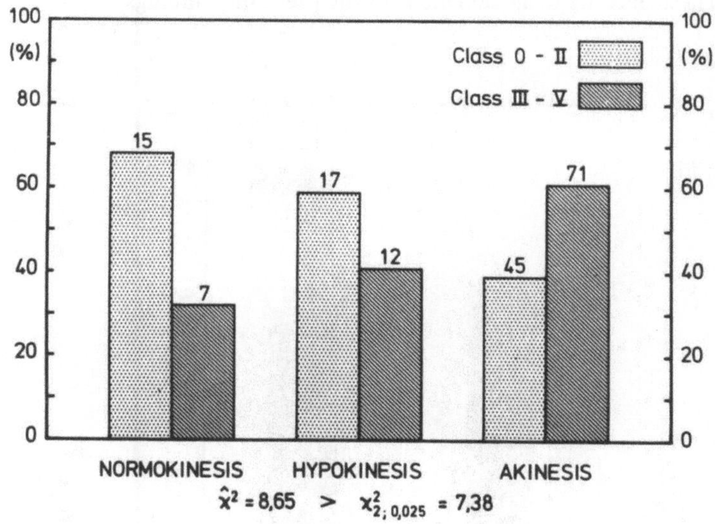

Fig. 4. b Maximal grading of *VES* in relation to left ventricular wall motion

(53) demonstrate high frequency of VES in comparison to only 14% (four patients) with hypokinetic and the same percentage of patients with normal wall motion ($P < 0.0005$).

The same close correlation is found between left ventricular wall motion abnormalities and maximal grading of VES. Figure 4b shows an increase in complex dysrhythmias classes III–V from 32% (seven patients) to 41% (12 patients) and finally to 61% (71 patients) with reduction of left ventricular motility. X^2 analysis confirms significant differences between the six groups ($P < 0.025$).

Akinetic left ventricular wall motion involved the anterior wall 70 times and the posterior wall 46 times. No relationship can be demonstrated between complex forms of VES and the site of akinetic regions, the significant grades III–V being equally represented in both locations, i.e., 63% (44 patients) and 59% (27 patients), respectively (Fig. 5). In conclusion, ischemic damage of the myocardium – independent of its location – seems to be a determining factor of ectopic activity.

Ectopic Activity in Relation to Left Ventricular Function

Since ischemic damage of the myocardium coincides more or less with impaired left ventricular function, an analogous relationship to hemodynamic findings should be expected. To prove this assumption, the maximal grading of VES according to Lown's definition was correlated with cardiac index, with ejection fraction, and with left ventricular enddiastolic pressure measured before and immediately after left ventricular angiography (Table 2). In fact, cardiac index and ejection fraction are significantly depressed and left ventricular enddiastolic pressure elevated in patients generating VES grades III–V in comparison with those showing ectopic activity classes 0–II. These data are in agreement with the preceding findings.

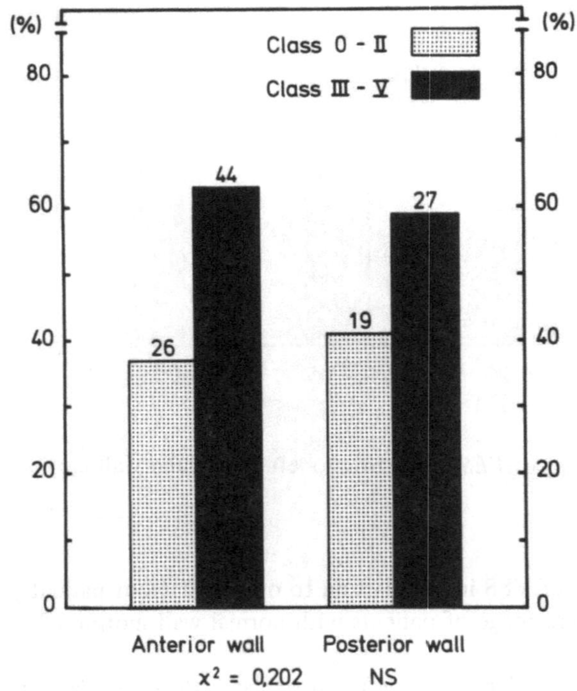

Fig. 5. Maximal grading of *VES* and localization of akinetic areas

Table 2. Maximal grade of VES and hemodynamic parameter

Lown class	CI (l/min/m²)		EF (%)		LVEDP (mm Hg) before angiography		after	
0–II	3.2	± 0.6	56.1	± 15.7	12.7	± 6.6	20.7	± 7.9
III–V	2.8	± 0.6	41.1	± 15.4	19.0	± 8.1	25.9	± 8.0
P	<0.005		<0.001		<0.001		<0.005	

Abbreviations: *CI*, cardiac index; *EF*, ejection fraction; *LVEDP*, left ventricular end-diastolic pressure

Conclusion and Clinical Implications

In conclusion, coronary patients with left ventricular akinetic wall motion – this predominantly implies patients *after* myocardial infarction – are prone not only to produce congestive heart failure but also life-threatening arrhythmias. In consequence, there is no contradiction between a history of recurrent congestive heart failure and sudden cardiac death due to electrical instability of the myocardium. But the post-event differentiation of sudden cardiac deaths due to dysrhythmias or due to pump failure, raises at times substantial difficulties.

References

1 Bethge K-P, Lichtlen PR (1979) Ventricular arrhythmias in relation to the extent of coronary lesions and left ventricular function. In: MacFarlane PW (ed) Progress in electrocardiology. Pitman Medical, Tunbridge Wells, pp 126–132

2 Bethge K-P, Bethge H-C, Lichtlen PR (1976) Häufigkeit von Kammer-Extrasystolen bei koronarer Herzkrankheit. Vergleich der Langzeit-EKG-Befunde mit der Koronarographie. Verh Dtsch Ges Kreislaufforsch 42:259

3 Bethge K-P, Bethge H-C, Graf A, van den Berg E, Lichtlen PR (1977) Kammer-Arrhythmien bei chronisch koronarer Herzkrankheit. Analyse anhand des Langzeit-Elektrokardiogrammes und der selektiven Koronarangiographie bzw. linksventrikulären Angiographie. Z Kardiol 66:1

4 Bruschke AVG, Proudfitt WL, Sones FM (1973) Progress study of 590 consecutive nonsurgical cases of coronary disease follwed 5–9 years. I. Arteriographic correlations. Circulation 47:1147

5 Bruschke AVG, Proudfitt WL, Sones FM (1973) Progress study of 590 consecutive nonsurgical cases of coronary disease followed 5–9 years. II. Ventriculographic and other correlations. Circulation 47:1154

6 Burggraf GW, Parker JO (1975) Prognosis in coronary artery disease. Angiographic, hemodynamic and clinical factors. Circulation 51:146

7 Calvert A, Lown B, Gorlin R (1977) Ventricular premature beats and anatomically defined coronary heart disease. Am J Cardiol 39:627

8 Chiang BN, Perlman LV, Ostrander LD, Epstein FH (1969) Relationship of premature systoles to coronary heart disease and sudden death in the Tecumseh epidemiologic study. Ann Intern Med 70:1159

9 The Coronary Drug Project Research Group (1973) Prognostic importance of premature beats followed myocardial infarction. JAMA 223:1116
10 Humphries J, O'N, Kuller L, Ross RS, Friesinger GC, Page EE (1974) Natural history of ischemic heart disease in relation to arteriographic findings. A twelve-year study of 224 patients. Circulation 49:489
11 Kotler MN, Tabatznik B, Mower MM, Tominaga S (1973) Prognostic significance of ventricular ectopic beats with respect to sudden death in the late postinfarction period. Circulation 47:959
12 Kühn P, Kroiss A, Joskowicz G (1976) Arrhythmieanalyse – Arrhythmieüberwachung. Vergleichsuntersuchungen von 4 Kleincomputern zur automatischen EKG-Überwachung. Z Kardiol 65:166
13 Lichtlen P (1979) Koronarangiographie und Prognose der koronaren Herzkrankheit. In: Lichtlen PR (ed) Koronarangiographie. Perimed, Erlangen, pp 375–385
14 Lown B, Wolf M (1971) Approaches to sudden death from coronary heart disease. Circulation 44:130
15 Moss AJ, Decamilla J, Engstrom F, Hoffmann W, Odoroff C, Davis H (1974) The posthospital phase of myocardial infarction: identification of patients with increased mortality risk. Circulation 49:460
16 Neilson JM (1974) High speed analysis of ventricular arrhythmias from 24 hour recordings. Computers in Cardiology, IEEE Catalogue No 74 CH 0379–7C, 55
17 Steinbrunn W, Lichtlen PR (1977) Complete 5-years accumulative survival rates in 244 unselected, unoperated coronary patients undergoing angiography. Circulation (Suppl III) 56:174
18 Tietze U, Leitner E-R v, Andresen D, Schröder R (1979) Ein Langzeit-EKG-Analysesystem zur quantitativen Auswertung von Herzrhythmusstörungen. Biomed Techn (Berlin) 24:275
19 Tietze U, Andresen D, Leitner E-R v, Schröder R (1979) Quantitative Auswertung von Langzeit-EKG-Registrierungen, Methode und Genauigkeit. Biomed Tech (Berlin) (Suppl 24):30
20 Van Durme JP, Pannier R (1978) Prevalence and prognostic significance of ventricular dysrrhythmias during the first year after myocardial infarction. In: Mäurer W, Schömig A, Dietz R, Lichtlen PR (eds) Betablockade 1977. Thieme, Stuttgart, pp 286–293
21 Vismara LA, Amsterdam EA, Mason DT (1975) Relation of ventricular arrhythmias in the late hospital phase of acute myocardial infarction to sudden death after hospital discharge. Am J Med 59:6
22 Webster JS, Moberg C, Rincon G (1974) Natural history of severe proximal coronary artery disease as documented by coronary cineangiography. Am J Cardiol 33:195

Part IV
Complementary Methods

Analysis of Drug Effects on Left Ventricular Isovolumic Contraction During Atrial Pacing

P.W. Serruys, R.W. Brower, J. Lubsen, M. v.d. Brand,
G.T. Meester, and P.G. Hugenholtz*

Introduction

The atrial pacing stress test has found application in the assessment of left ventricular function [1, 3, 12, 13, 15, 18, 20, 28], but the usefulness of this procedure in the assessment of drug effects on left ventricular function has still to be demonstrated [6, 7, 9, 11, 14].

Global and regional left ventricular function in patients with coronary artery disease is often normal at rest and is only impaired during stress, when transient regional asynergy is provoked by a localized imbalance between oxygen supply and demand. Therefore, the effects of an antianginal drug or an antiarrhythmic agent or even an inotropic drug should be studied not only under resting conditions, but also under a stress situation.

In the evaluation of ventricular function in patients with coronary artery disease, the atrial pacing stress test (APST) is attractive for a number of methodological reasons: first, the test can be applied to patients at rest, thus obviating any unwanted systematic change due to muscular exercise, and second, the stress, increased heart rate, can be controlled exactly both in duration and in magnitude.

To be of value, the test and the measurements on which it is based should have good reproducibility relative to the effect of the medication [27]. Having demonstrated the reproducibility of this test, we show that the APST can be used in quick succession to measure the effects of drugs. Data on two drugs which have been studied are given as examples. The first one is a potent antiarrhythmic agent suspected of having a negative inotropic effect. The second is a calcium antagonist, which is also supposed to have negative inotropic properties.

Methods

The APST is performed by pacing the right atrium from resting heart rate to the highest rate in steps of ten beats per minute while simultaneously measuring the pressure-derived variables with a dual tip manometer (Fig. 1).

Patients are studied after an overnight fast without premedication. Beta blockade is withdrawn at least 24 h prior to catheterization. Following right heart catheterization and measurement of cardiac output (thermodilution method) a bipolar pacing electrode

---

* With the technical assistance of Ms. I. Zorn

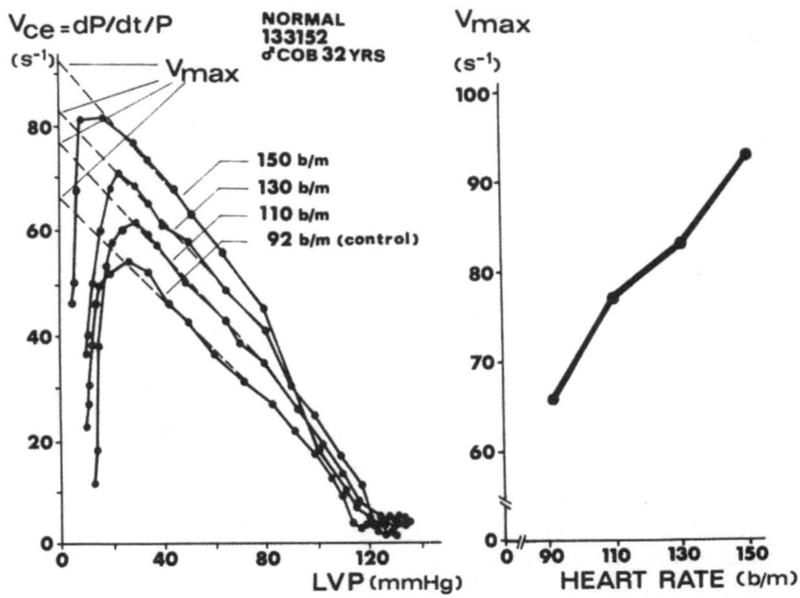

Fig. 1. Progressive deviation of the *dP/dt* on *P* curve during atrial pacing at increasing heart rate. In this normal subject, *Vmax* increases from 65 to 95 s^{-1} during pacing-induced tachycardia

catheter is positioned high in the right atrium. The left ventricle is catheterized via a right brachial arteriotomy and pressures are recorded by a Millar Instruments 7F dual tip manometer catheter. The reference level is set at mid-chest and compared with the fluid channel for base line correction.

After control determinations of left ventricular pressure, the APST is started at a level just above control heart rate. One to two min is allowed for stabilization followed by a 20 s data acquisition period where at least 12 heart beats are processed and averaged using the representative beat method [16, 26] (Fig. 2). The pacing rate is then increased in steps of 10 to 20 bpm and the measurements repeated. Pacing is continued until (1) a rate of 180 bpm; (2) the onset of chest pain; or (3) A-V dissociation occurred or recurring extrasystoles made the interpretation of the results doubtful. Angiography follows the APST.

During the APST the following left ventricular pressure (P) derived variables were determined:

1. Peak LV systolic pressure (LVSP, mm Hg);
2. LV enddiastolic pressure (LVEDP, mm Hg);
3. Peak positive first derivative of LV pressure (Pk dP/dt, mm Hg/s);
4. Peak LV dP/dt/P from total pressure providing $P > 20$ mm Hg (Pk Vce, s^{-1});
5. dP/dt/P at 40 mm Hg total pressure (Vce (40), s^{-1});
6. dP/dt/P extrapolated to $P = 0$ mm Hg total pressure using a linear least squares fit from peak dP/dt/P to begin ejection (Vmax, s^{-1})

```
ID:      12981                    105 | 27-MAR-80
NR:  80-0229  C:  0  R:   97  F:24:25 |  10:44:30
```

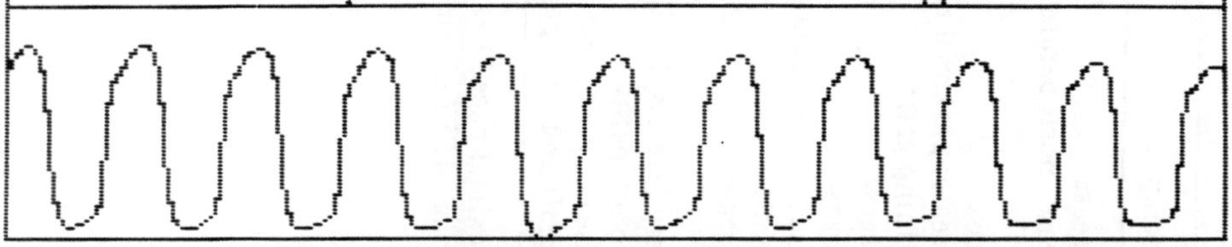

HRATE	LVEDP	PKSYS	DP/DT	PKVCE	TVMAX	-DP/DT
92	15	162	2233	49.2	63.2	2788
100	10	152	2195	60.8	69.1	2599
110	8	148	2310	70.7	76.2	2706
120	6	148	2399	72.7	79.2	2737
129	7	144	2443	66.3	75.4	2885
139	5	154	2663	78.5	84.5	3028
150	2	138	2544	78.2	87.3	2744
160	2	144	2920	81.6	94.5	3227
98	20	168	2541	45.6	66.4	2850

Fig. 2. After each increment in heart rate, 1 min is allowed for stabilization, followed by a 20 s data acquisition period where at least 12 heart beats are processed and averaged using the representative beat method of Stenson. Pacing is continued until a rate of 180 bpm is reached, unless onset of chest pain or atrioventricular dissociation occurs, prior to this rate

Reproducibility of Hemodynamic Parameters During Pacing Stress Test

To assess the reproducibility of our method, an atrial pacing stress test was carried out twice in ten patients with proven coronary artery disease. Five of them experienced angina during both tests (Table 1). The time interval between the tests was 20 min.

From the duplicate measurements at each level of heart rate, the standard deviations (sd) of the random error component (e) in the measurements were estimated by:

$$sd(e) = \sqrt{\frac{\sum_{i=1}^{N} \left(n_i \sum_{j=i}^{ni} \frac{dij^2}{2n_i} \right)}{\sum_{i=1}^{N} ni}}$$

where: N = number of patients, i.e., ten

n_i = number of measurements made during the APSTs of the i-th patient

d_{ij} = the j-th difference between the first and the second APST measurement at a given heart rate for the i-th patient.

Table 1. Patient data: Group studied for assessment of the reproducibility of the atrial pacing stress test (APST)

Patient	Age	Sex	NYHA	EF %	EDV ml/m^2	APST$_1$	APST$_2$	Coronary angiography
1. C.V.	47	M	III	0.26	118	160 – *AP*	160 – AP	Three-vessel disease
2. G.O.	46	M	I	0.66	71	170 – AV	170 – AV	One-vessel disease; postoperative one patient graft
3. A.L.	46	M	II	0.55	96	180 – *AP*	180 – AP	One-vessel disease
4. C.K.	60	M	III	0.56	92	120 – AP – LBBB	120 – AP – LBBB	Three-vessel disease; proximal narrowing (75%). Jump graft
5. J.M.H.	50	M	II	0.68	69	120 – *AP*	120 – AP	Three-vessel disease
6. J.H.	53	M	II	0.44	113	120 – AVB	120 – AVB	Three-vessel disease
7. J.B.	62	M	II	0.65	79	170 – AVB	170 – AVB	Three-vessel disease; postoperative one occluded graft
8. C.D.V.	55	F	III	0.56	77	120 – *AP*; 150 – AVB	120 – AP; 150 – AVB	Three-vessel disease
9. A.H.B.	42	M	II	0.73	68	150 – AVB	150 – AVB	Normal coronary arteries, LV biopsy; incipiens cardiomyopathy
10. L.V.A.	42	M	II	0.68	57	150 – AVB	150 – AVB	Three-vessel disease; postoperative one occluded graft and one open graft

Abbreviations: NYHA, functional class; *EF*, ejection fraction (%); *EDV*, enddiastolic volumes (ml/m^2); $APST_1$, maximal paced heart rate (bpm) and cause of arrest (*AP*, onset of angina pectoris; *AVB*, atrioventricular block); during the first atrial pacing; $APST_2$, same data during the second atrial pacing

Sd (e) is a parameter which describes the spread of the measurements if they were repeated while the actual value remained constant. It is the "yardstick" of the reproducibility of a measurement. Equation 1 is a weighted average of a well-known estimator of sd (e) when duplicate measurements are available [2].

The duplicate measurements obtained during two consecutive APSTs are presented in Fig. 3. Sd (e) was estimated as 6.0 mm Hg for LVP, 1.9 mm Hg for EDP and 3.0 s^{-1} for Vmax respectively. In addition, for none of these parameters does the random error seem to depend on heart rate (Fig. 4).

In Fig. 4 are plotted the differences between two consecutive measurements versus heart rate. The differences observed in left ventricular pressure, enddiastolic pressure and Vmax during the two consecutive measurements are not affected by the increase

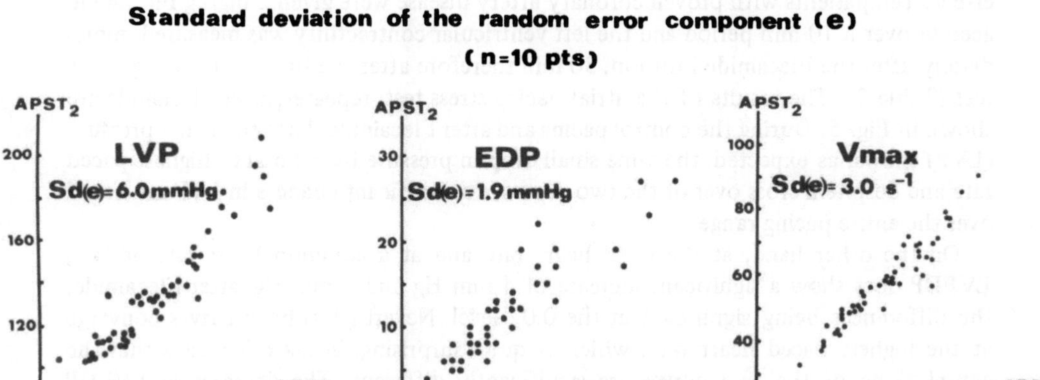

Fig. 3. Reproducibility of the atrial pacing stress test (*APST*). Standard deviation (*Sd*) of the random error component (*e*). *LVP*, left ventricular pressure; *EDP*, enddiastolic pressure

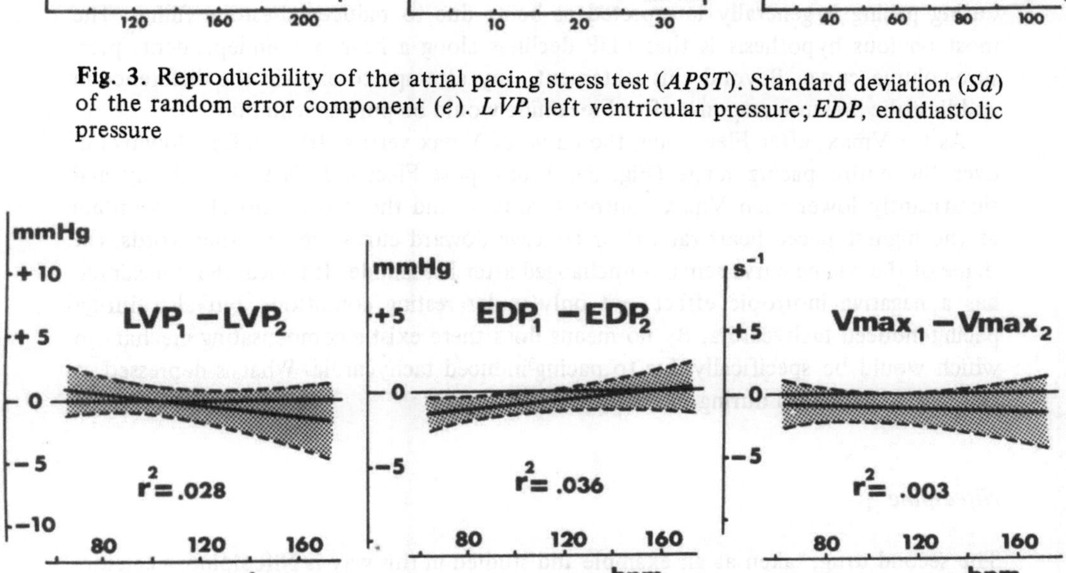

Fig. 4. Differences in *LVP, EDP,* and *Vmax* versus heart rate during two consecutive atrial pacing stress tests (*$APST_1$* and *$APST_2$*)

in heart rate, so that the average differences between the two measurements remain close to zero over the entire pacing range.

Therefore, it is concluded that these measurements made during an APST have excellent reproducibility and that the APST can be used in quick succession to test the action of drugs.

Drug Studies

Flecainide Acetate

This type of analysis was applied to two different drugs. The first one – Flecainide acetate – is a potent anti-arrhythmic agent, suspected of having a negative inotropic effect. Ten patients with proven coronary artery disease were given 2 mg/kg Flecainide acetate over a 10 min period and the left ventricular contractility was measured immediately after the Flecainide infusion, 30 min therefore after the first atrial pacing stress test (Table 2). The results of the atrial pacing stress test, repeated after Flecainide are shown in Fig. 5. During the control pacing and after Flecainide, left ventricular pressure (LVP) shows, as expected, the same small drop in pressure from basal to highest paced rate and despite a cross over of the two curves, no significant changes in LVP are noted over the entire pacing range.

On the other hand, at the basal heart rate and at a common heart rate of 100, LVEDP does show a significant increase of 4 mm Hg and 2 mm Hg, after Flecainide, the differences being significant at the 0.02 level. Nevertheless both curves converge at the highest paced heart rate, which is quite surprising, because it means that the actual slope of the two curves are significantly different. The decrease in LVEDP during pacing is generally interpreted as being due to reduced diastolic filling. The most obvious hypothesis is that EDP declines along a heart rate-independent, pressure-volume curve. Beyond this statement, any attempt to explain the difference in enddiastolic pressure response after Flecainide would be pure speculation.

As for Vmax, after Flecainide, the curve of Vmax versus HR is shifted downward, over the entire pacing range (Fig. 5). Vmax post Flecainide is systematically and significantly lower than Vmax control (Table 3) and the two relationships maintain at the highest paced heart rate, their concave doward curvature. In other words, the shape of the pacing curve remains unchanged after Flecainide. It is clear that Flecainide has a negative inotropic effect, not only under resting conditions, but also during pacing-induced tachycardia. By no means does there exist a compensating mechanism which would be specifically due to pacing-induced tachycardia. What is depressed at rest, is also depressed during the stress test.

Nifedipine

The second drug, taken as an example and studied in this way is Nifedipine, a calcium antagonist, which basically is supposed to have negative inotropic properties [10, 21, 22, 24]. A group of 11 patients (all males) received intravenous injections of Nifedipine 1 year after coronary bypass grafting. Nine were in NYHA function class I and two in

Table 2. Patient material for the Flecainide study

Patient	Age	Sex	NYHA	EF %	EDV ml/m^2	APST$_1$ Control	APST$_2$ Flecainide	Coronary angiography
1. J.N.D.	55	M	II	0.52	88	160 – AP	140 – AVB	Three-vessel disease
2. C.J.	45	M	II	0.61	82	150 – AVB	120 – AVB	Three-vessel disease
3. A.G.J.	52	M	III	0.54	71	140 – AP	120 – AP	Three-vessel disease
4. J.B.	52	M	II	0.61	58	140 – AVB	130 – AVB	Two-vessel disease
5. J.M.G.D.	52	M	III	0.56	75	120 – AP	120 – AP	Three-vessel disease
6. K.M.	58	M	II	0.63	43	130 – AVB	120 – AVB	Three-vessel disease; postoperative one patient graft and one occluded graft
7. L.G.	52	M	III	0.62	72	140 – AP	140 – AVB	Three-vessel disease
8. J.D.G.	60	M	II	0.37	94	140 – AP	140 – LBBB	One-vessel disease
9. J.W.W.	58	F	II	0.62	47	140 – AP	140 – VT + AP	Two-vessel disease
10. J.H.B.	36	F	II	–	81	180 – AVB	160 – AVB	Normal coronary angiogram

Same abbreviations as in Table 1. *VT*, ventricular tachycardia

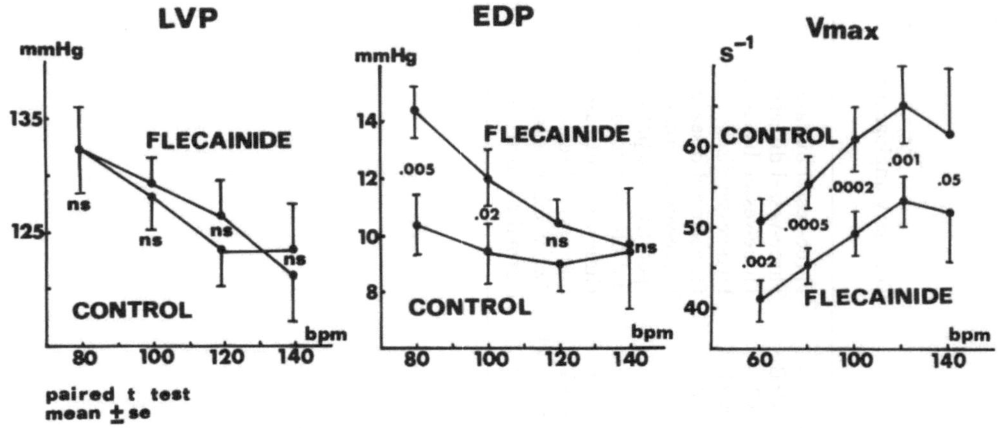

Fig. 5. Peak systolic pressure (*LVP*), left ventricular enddiastolic pressure (*EDP*), and *Vmax* (control versus Flecainide, mean ± SEM) at basal heart rate and during pacing-incuded tachycardia

class II (Table 4). There was no occurrence of precordial pain during the control pacing and during the test after Nifedipine. The heart rates terminating the atrial pacing stress tests were precisely the same for each patient during the control stress test and the Nifedipine stress test. After the control pacing test, we waited 20 min and monitored the pressure-derived variables until they returned to control values. An intravenous (iv) infusion of 1 mg Nifedipine was performed over 3 min. All tests and measurements were repeated starting 3 min after endinfusion. The atrial pacing stress test after Nifedipine was performed in the same way as during the control determinations. During pacing-induced tachycardia after Nifedipine, peak LVP remained 100 mm Hg below control values at both a common heart rate of 120 bpm and at the highest rate (147 bpm at control, 148 bpm Nifedipine).

Enddiastolic pressure (EDP) showed no significant change at a common heart rate of 120 (10 vs 10.5 mm Hg), but during the control pacing we observed an increase at the highest pacing rate (Fig. 6) which represents a compromised response [13]. After Nifedipine this increase disappeared and instead the normal decrease in EDP was observed. Nevertheless, this response cannot be considered as completely normal because of the slightly elevated basal values, but rather as an improved response. After Nifedipine there was a decrease in EDP at the highest paced rate from 11.2 to 7.4 mm Hg ($P < 0.05$), so that the negative slope of EDP vs heart rate increased from 0.095 to 0.190 mm Hg/bpm ($P < 0.02$).

Vmax at basal heart rate and at a common heart rate of 120 was unchanged, however at the highest paced rate the trend of Vmax to increase (61 s^{-1} C vs 68 s^{-1} N) after Nifedipine became significant at the 0.02 level (Fig. 7). This confirms previous findings that Nifedipine at a therapeutic dose appears to have no negative inotropic effect. Indeed, possibly a slight positive inotropic effect is observed.

In these patients 29 radiopaque epicardial marker pairs had been implanted during surgery and a total of 26 bypasses had been grafted of which 23 remained patent 1 year after surgery [4, 5, 23, 25]. Two marker pairs were located in regions with occluded

Table 3. Velocities of the contractile element (VCE) during pacing-induced tachycardia (control versus Flecainide, mean ± SEM) Student's t-test for paired data. *TP*, total pressure; *DP*, developed pressure

		80 bpm	P value	100 bpm	P value	120 bpm	P value
VCE 40 s^{-1}	Control	36 ± 1.6	5.10^{-4}	41 ± 2.5	5.10^{-4}	44 ± 3.3	0.002
	Flecainide	30 ± 1.3		33 ± 2.1		36 ± 2.2	
Pk VCE 40 s^{-1}	Control	46 ± 3.6	5.10^{-4}	52 ± 3.6	5.10^{-4}	56 ± 5	0.001
	Flecainide	36 ± 3.1		42 ± 3.1		46 ± 3.5	
Vmax TP s^{-1}	Control	56 ± 2.5	5.10^{-4}	61 ± 3.8	2.10^{-4}	66 ± 4.8	0.001
	Flecainide	46 ± 1.9		50 ± 3.1		54 ± 3.3	
Vmax s^{-1}	Control	77 ± 4.4	0.005	84 ± 4.8	0.002	90 ± 5.4	2.10^{-4}
	Flecainide	68 ± 3.1		71 ± 3.6		74 ± 3.6	

Table 4. Summary of the patient material for the nifedipine study

Age	Sex	Preop (NYHA)	Postop (NYHA)	Subjective change	Comments	EF	EDV ml/m^2
46	M	II	I	Cured	Previous inferior MI	0.54	68
48	M	II	I	Cured	Previous inferior MI	0.54	56
45	M	III	I	Cured	LV hypertrophy	–	–
56	M	III	II	Improved	–	0.75	52
62	M	II–III	II	Improved	Previous inferior and anterolateral MI	0.50	90
45	M	II	I	Cured	Previous anterior-inferior MI	0.39	102
48	M	II	I	Cured	Previous small anteroseptal MI	–	59
51	M	II–III	I	Cured	Previous anterior and inferior MI, possible LVH	0.69	77
59	M	II	I	Cured	Previous inferior MI	0.57	72
63	M	II–III	I	Cured	Previous anterioseptal MI	0.34	88
60	M	II–III	I	Cured	Previous inferior and anterior MI	0.66	95

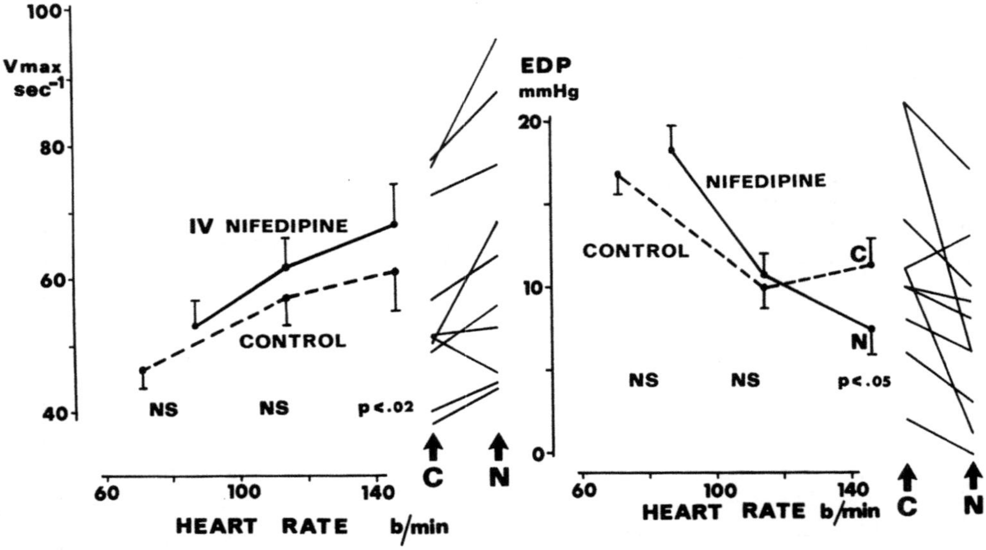

Fig. 6. Peak systolic pressure (*LVP*), left ventricular enddiastolic pressure (*EDP*), and *Vmax* from total pressure (control versus Nifedipine, mean ± SEM) at basal heart rate and during pacing-induced tachycardia. *Right*, individual patient plots of *EDP* and *Vmax* at the highest paced heart rate

bypasses. One of them (occluded graft and patent coronary artery), showed a paradoxical systolic expansion during the control atrial pacing. As shown in Fig. 8, at a heart rate of 120 bpm, the unsuccessfully bypassed region becomes dyskinetic, exhibiting a paradoxical systolic expansion and VCE 40 drops from 27.2 s^{-1} to 23.2 s^{-1}. After Nifedipine, a higher level of stress (140 bpm) could have been reached before the segmental dysfunction becomes apparent and before the drop of the isovolumic indices.

This peculiar observation gives us some insight into the mechanism of action of the drug.

It has been shown recently that regional coronary blood flow after Nifedipine is increased during pacing-induced tachycardia, even in the poststenotic coronary segment [8]. From an increase in flow in an underperfused and ischemic area we can expect an improvement in regional wall motion, under a stress situation.

In this particular case, the postNifedipine increase in Vmax during pacing could be explained by the anti-ischemic properties of the drug.

Discussion and Conclusion

The reason for considering the APST as a pertinent factor in the evaluation of drugs in patients with CAD is that there may be beneficial or detrimental effects of the drug which are not apparent at basal heart rate.

The effects of an increase in heart rate on Vmax before and after Nifedipine, and before and after Flecainide are shown in Fig. 7. For Nifedipine, the difference between

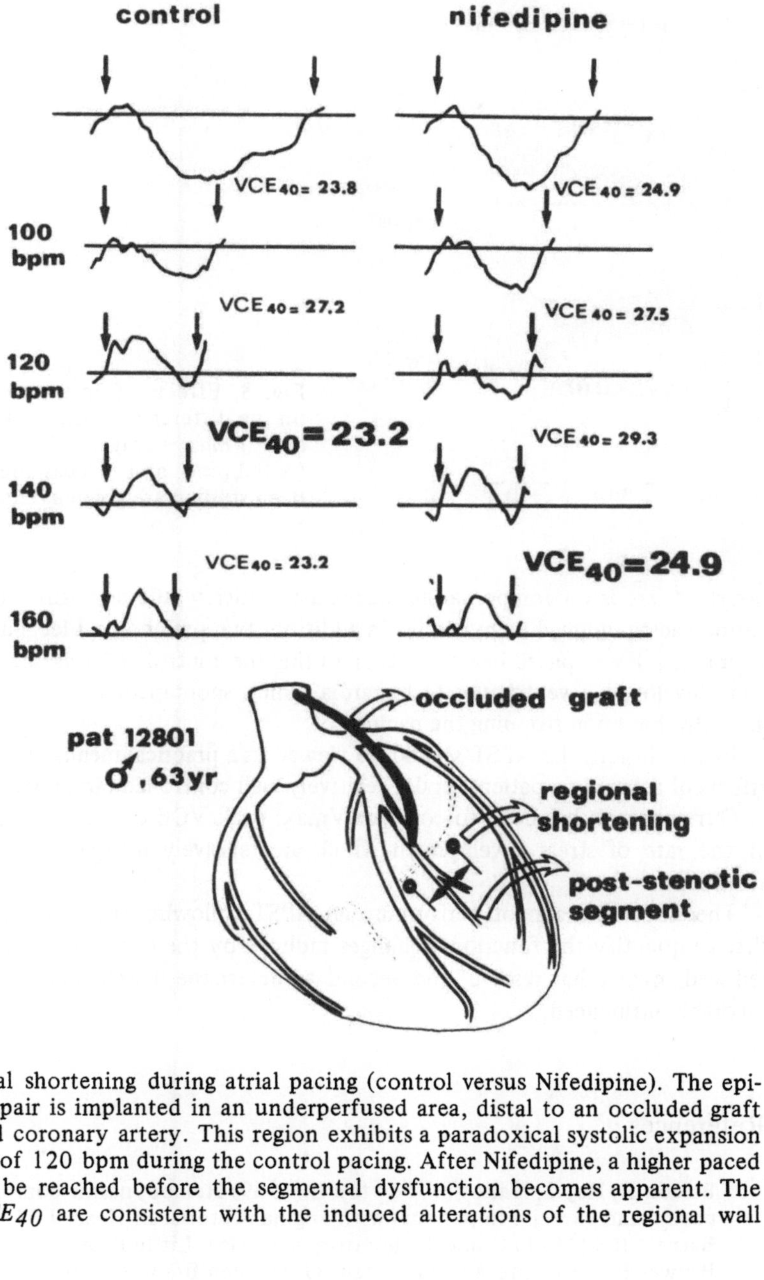

Fig. 7. Regional shortening during atrial pacing (control versus Nifedipine). The epicardial marker pair is implanted in an underperfused area, distal to an occluded graft and a narrowed coronary artery. This region exhibits a paradoxical systolic expansion at a heart rate of 120 bpm during the control pacing. After Nifedipine, a higher paced heart rate can be reached before the segmental dysfunction becomes apparent. The changes in VCE_{40} are consistent with the induced alterations of the regional wall motion

Vmax (control) and Vmax (drug) increases progressively with the increase in heart rate. In other words, a beneficial effect does appear, but only at the highest paced rate. This is supported by recent metabolic studies which have shown that pacing-induced ischemia can be reversed by Nifedipine [17].

Conversely, for Flecainide, despite a nonsignificant coefficient of correlation, it appears that Vmax after Flecainide is decreased mostly at the highest paced rate. Ob-

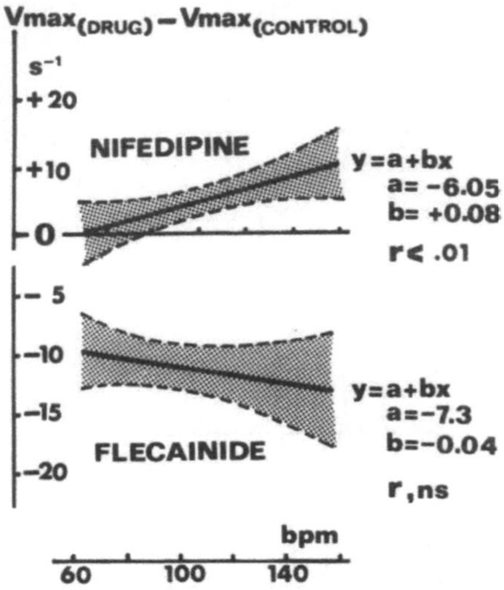

Fig. 8. Effects of an increase in heart rate on the differences between *Vmax* (controls) and *Vmax* (drugs). Data on two drugs (Nifedipine and Flecainide) which have been studied are given as examples

viously, there is no compensating mechanism which would normalize the contractility during pacing-induced tachycardia. In addition, two patients on Flecainide experienced angina at a lower paced heart rate than during the control atrial pacing stress test. One even developed a ventricular tachycardia which spontaneously reverted to a normal sinus rhythm upon stopping the pacing.

In conclusion, the APST should be viewed as a practical means of stress-testing the effects of a drug in a patient, under relatively well controlled circumstances.

Our approach has been to consider Vmax, peak VCE etc., as normalized measures of the rate of stress development which are relatively independent of preload and afterload.

Therefore, the aim of performing an APST following the drug administration is first to quantify the functional changes induced by the drug, in terms of improved or reduced myocardial reserve, and second to determine if ischemia is favorably or unfavorably influenced.

References

1 Balcon R, Hay J, Malloy W, Sowton E (1969) Hemodynamic comparisons of atrial pacing and exercise in patients with angina pectoris. Br Heart J 31:168

2 Barnett RN (1971) Clinical laboratory statistica. Little Brown, Boston, p 84

3 Brower RW, Remme WJ, ten Katen HJ, van den Brand M (1977) Quantification of atrial pacing stress test: normal values and limits between normal and abnormal for coronary artery disease in man. Comput Cardiol, pp 591–599

4 Brower RW, ten Katen HJ, Meester GT (1978) A method for determining regional shortening from radiopaque markers in man after bypass surgery. Am J Cardiol 41:1222

5 Brower RW, Serruys PW, Bos E, Nauta J (1979) Bypass flow, reactive hyperemia and regional myocardial shortening after coronary artery bypass surgery. J Thorac Cardiovasc Surg 77:92–100

6 Chiong MA, West RO, Parker JO (1972) Influence of nitroglycerin on myocardial metabolism and hemodynamics during angina induced by atrial pacing. Circulation 45:1044
7 Chiong MA, West RO, Parker JO (1976) The protective effect of glucose-insulin-potassium on the response to atrial pacing. Circulation 54:37
8 Engel HJ, Lichtlen PR (1980) Regional myocardial blood supply to the normal and poststenotic ischemic areas after nifedipine. In: Puech P, Krebs R (eds) 4th international Adalat symposium 1979. Excerpta Medica, Amsterdam
9 Erick MJ, Balcon R, Cross D, Sowton E (1968) Hemodynamic effects of nitroglycerin in patients with angina pectoris studied by an atrial pacing method. Circulation 37:160
10 Fleckenstein A, Tritthart H, Döring HJ, Byon KY (1972) Bay a 1040 – ein hochaktiver Ca^{++} – antagonistischer Inhibitor der elektromechanischen Koppelungsprozesse im Warmblüter-Myokard. Arzneim Forsch 22:22
11 Helfant RH, Forrester JS, Hampton JR, Haft JI, Kemp HG, Gorlin R (1970) Differential hemodynamic metabolic and electrocardiographic effects in subjects with and without angina pectoris during atrial pacing. Circulation 42:602
12 Hugenholtz PG, Roelandt JR, Brower R (1975) Myocardial muscle performance in coronary artery disease. In: Bess P, Bricaud H (eds) Performance ventriculaire chez l'homme. Expansion scientifique, Paris, p 403
13 Hugenholtz PG, Meester GT, van den Brand M, Brower RW, ten Katen HJ, Bos E (1977) Pre and post operative evaluation of left ventricular function after coronary bypass grafting. In: Yu PN, Goodwin JF (eds) Progress in cardiology. Lea & Febiger, Philadelphia, p 165–183
14 Jackson G, Atkinson L, Aram S (1977) Improvement of myocardial metabolism in coronary arterial disease by beta-blockade. Br Heart J 39:829
15 Linhart JW, Hildner FJ, Barold S, Lister JW, Samet P (1969) Left hemodynamics during angina pectoris induced by atrial pacing. Circulation 40:483
16 Meester GI, Bernard N, Zeelenberg C, Brower RW, Hugenholtz PG (1975) A computer system for real time analysis of cardiac catheterization data. Cathet Cardiovasc Diagn 1:113
17 Merillon JP, Morgant C, Zygelman M, Beaufils Ph, Patart O, Chapuy JY, Gourgon R (1978) Comparison des effects hemodynamiques et coronariens de deux drogues vasodilatatrices anti-angineuses: la Nifedipine et la Trinitrine. Arch Mal Coeur 17: 913
18 O'Brien KP, Higgs LM, Glancy DL, Epstein SE (1969) Hemodynamic accompaniments of angina. A comparison during angina induced by exercise and by atrial pacing. Circulation 39:735
19 Parker JO, Chiong MA, West RO, Case RB (1969) Sequential alterations in myocardial lactate metabolism, S-T segments, and left ventricular function during angina induced by atrial pacing. Circulation 40:113
20 Parker JO, Ledwick JR, West RO, Case RB (1969) Reversible cardiac failure during angina pectoris. Hemodynamic effects of atrial pacing in coronary artery disease. Circulation 39:745
21 Raff KH, Kosche F, Lockner W (1972) Untersuchungen mit Nifedipine, einer coronargefäßerweiternden Substanz mit schneller sublingualer Wirkung. Arzneim Forsch 22:33
22 Serruys PW, van den Brand M (1979) Effects of nifedipine on left ventricular isovolumic contraction following intravenous or intracoronary administration. Circulation (Suppl II) 59–60:82
23 Serruys PW, Hugenholtz PG, ten Katen HJ, Brower RW (1979) Effect of Nifedipine on regional ventricular shortening during pacing after coronary artery bypass grafting. In: Lichtlen P (ed) International Adalat Panel Discussion, new experimental and clinical results. Excerpta Medica, Amsterdam

24 Serruys PW, Brower RW, Bom AH, ten Katen HJ, Hugenholtz PG (1979) Contractility relaxation and regional wall motion following intracoronary injection of a Ca^{++} antagonist. Circulation (Suppl II) 59–60:180
25 Serruys PW, Brower RW, ten Katen HJ, van den Brand M, Hugenholtz PG (1979) Early myocardial depression after coronary artery bypass surgery. In: Roskam H, Schmuziger M (eds) Coronary heart surgery, a rehabilitation measure. Springer, Berlin Heidelberg New York, p 348
26 Stenson RE, Crouse L, Henry WL, Harrison DC (1978) A time shared digital computer system for on line analysis of cardiac catheterization data. Comput Biomed Research 1:605
27 Thadani U, Lewis JR, Mathew TM, West RO, Parker JO (1979) Reproducibility of clinical and hemodynamic parameters during pacing stress testing in patients with angina pectoris. Circulation 60:1036
28 Thadani U, Lewis RJ, West RO, Parker JO (1979) Clinical and hemodynamic responses during pacing in the supine and upright posture in angina pectoris. Am J Cardiol 44:249

Interest of Gamma-Angiocardiography at Rest, After Leg Raising, and After Nitroglycerin in Coronary Artery Disease and Myocardial Infarction

M. Brochier, T. Planiol, R. Itti, B. Charbonnier, P. Raynaud, and J. Helias

Introduction

The assessment of overall and regional ventricular disturbances in coronary artery disease (CAD) was performed with radionuclide angiography at rest [8], during a volume load leg raising test (LR) [4], then after an unloading nitroclycerin injection (NG) [5, 7, 10].

Material and Methods

One hundred patients were studied: 10 control people (group I), 25 with documented angina pectoris (group II), 27 with an acute myocardial infarction (AMI, group III), and 38 with an older myocardial infarction (OMI, group IV). All the patients underwent myocardial scintigraphy. Gamma-angiocardiography was performed at rest in the right anterior oblique view (RAO) at the first pass [11], then in frontal (FA) and in left anterior oblique views (LAO) at equilibrium [1, 2]. In 72 patients, another recording was obtained during stress consisting of LR to about 45 cm, during 3 min [4]. In 51 patients, a final recording was assessed after a slow intravenous injection of 1.5 mg NG in LAO or FA view according to the previous area of interest.

During both tests, continuous ECG and blood pressure were checked. The whole session was performed with a single intravenous injection of 20 mCi technetium-labeled serum albumin [3]. In each measurement, the studied parameters were the overall ejection fraction (GEF), the functional imaging and representative histograms (which give an EF point by point), then a regional ejection analysis with quantitative evaluation (REF) using hemiaxis technique and comparing the regional functional imaging and histograms. Finally, a qualitative study of left ventricular isocontours to assess asynergic segments (hypokinesis, akinesis, and dyskinesis) was performed. The changes of GEF and REF were considered as significative if the differences between at rest and after test parameters were at least 10%.

Correlations were established between these data and ECG disturbances (all cases) and coronary angiograms obtained in 35 patients: 17 of group II, 8 of group III, and 10 of group IV. In a prior study [9], as in many others, a good correlation had been found between ejection fraction estimates obtained by ECG-gated ventriculography and by biplane ventriculography ($r = 0.85$) and also between EF estimates obtained at first pass and at equilibrium.

Results

Group I: global and regional parameters of the left ventricular function, in normal subjects, tend to increase as well after LR test as after NG.

Group II: coronary heart disease without myocardial infarctions (Figs. 1, 2).

After LR test, the GEF does not decrease significantly. The regional EF and wall motion remain stable in 70% of cases. They increase in 19% and decrease in 11% of cases. Asynergic segments can appear which were not evident in recording at rest.

After NG infusion, the GEF increases significantly in 29% of cases. The REF and regional kinetic parameters increase in 43% of cases.

Group III: acute myocardial infarction (Figs. 1, 2).

After LR test: regional wall motion abnormalities appear to increase in 42% of cases, while they decrease in 29% of cases and remain unchanged in 29% of cases.

After NG infusion: the GEF and regional parameters improve respectively in 29% and in 62% of cases, remain stable in 24%, and worsen in 14% of cases.

Group IV: old myocardial infarctions (Figs. 1, 2).

After LR test, GEF decreases significantly in 23% of cases, RWM abnormalities worsen in 65% of cases, remain unchanged in 31%, and decrease in 4% of cases.

After NG: GEF improves significantly in 56% of cases. Local left ventricular parameters improve in 47% of cases, while they remain unmodified in 37%, and worsen in 16% of cases.

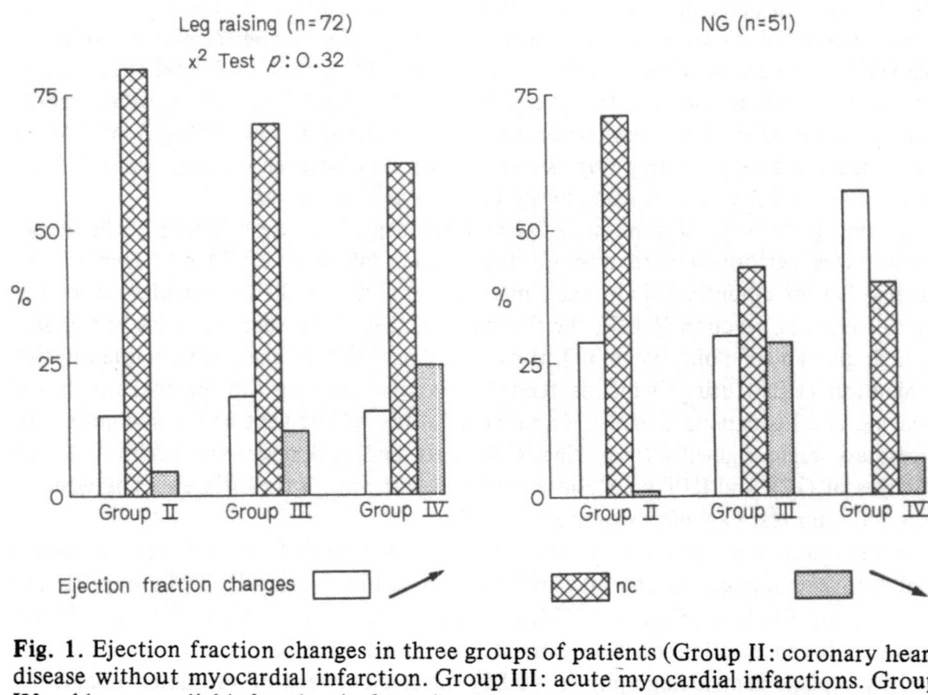

Fig. 1. Ejection fraction changes in three groups of patients (Group II: coronary heart disease without myocardial infarction. Group III: acute myocardial infarctions. Group IV: old myocardial infarctions) after a leg-raising test and after nitroglycerin injection) ↗, increase; *nc*, no change; ↘, decrease

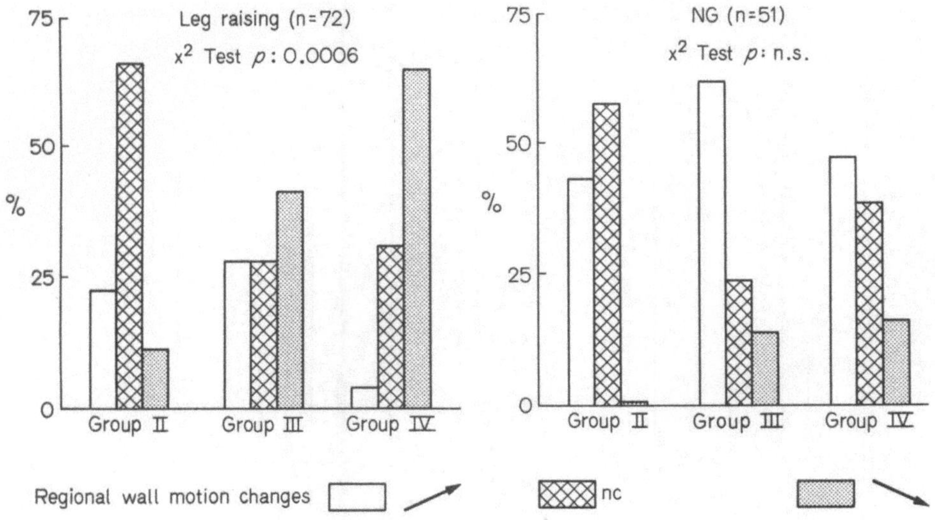

Fig. 2. Regional wall motion changes in the same three groups of patients as above

Thus, in the three groups of CAD, the GEF changes are poor after a loading LR test as well as after an unloading NG infusion (Fig. 3). However, LR test tends to impair the regional left ventricular function while NG infusion improves it and these changes are significant. The most dramatic changes are observed in groups III and IV (Fig. 2). The correlations with ECG and coronary angiograms demonstrate that impairment concerns the necrotic or injured areas.

Comments

With regard to the LR test, the method is quite benign, no incident occurring during the test, even in the group of AMI. Cardiac frequency and arterial blood pressure remained stable during and after LR. The test induces a noticeable increase in the preload and a slight increase in the postload. It can detect regional abnormalities of the ventricular function which did not appear in the radionuclide ventriculography at rest [4]. It is particularly useful to observe these data in the acute phase of myocardial infarction when X-ray ventriculography is not feasible [3]. But the LR test is less sensitive than the exertional test. It is of poor interest in stable angina.

Concerning the NG injection, no accident was observed during the unloading NG administration. However, important changes in arterial blood pressure occurred occasionally (a systolic pression decrease of 30 mm Hg on average), particularly in four cases of group III, related to a low filling defect. A lower dose of NG could be infused and eventual hypovolemia should be corrected before the test [6].

This test is not of the same interest according to the group of patients. In the group of CAD with no infarction, it can foresee the improvement that can be hoped for after a coronary bypass, if the improvement of RWM and parameters is recorded in the post-stenotic areas during the test [5].

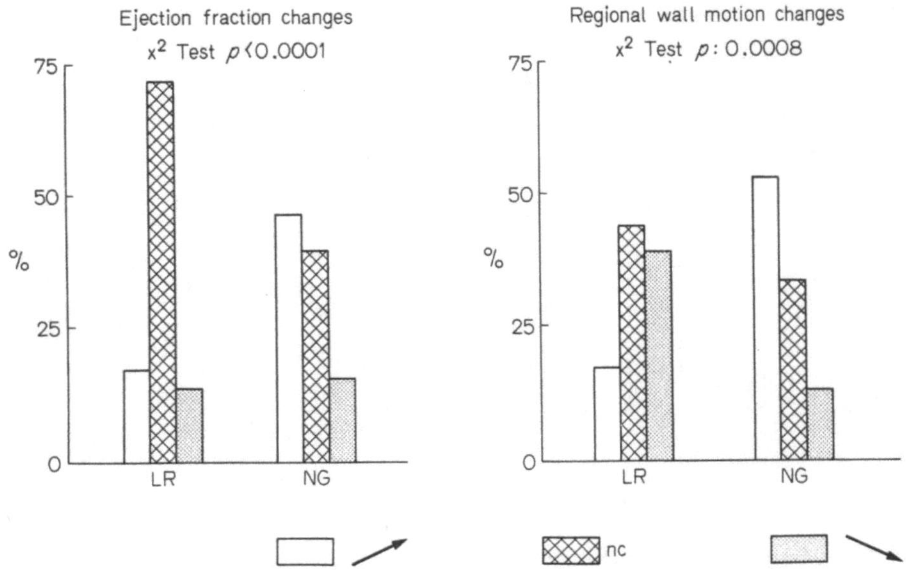

Fig. 3. Comparison between the effects of a leg-raising test (*LR*) and nitroglycerin injection (*NG*) on ejection fraction (*EE*) and regional wall motion (*RWM*) in coronary artery disease (*C.A.D.*); n = 123

In the group of AMI this test is available, after measurement of pulmonary capillary flow, to decide if vasodilators are advisable and also to detect the viable myocardial areas in the surrounding necrotic areas.

In the group of OMI, the test has advantages for both the second and third groups of CAD.

To conclude, GEF is the most important global parameter of the left ventricular function at rest [8], but it is not very sensitive in appreciating the changes after left ventricular loading or unloading tests [10]. On the contrary, regional EF or RWM modifications can be qualitatively and quantitatively assessed after a loading LR test and after an unloading NG infusion [5, 7, 10]. Both techniques are easily performed using radionuclide ventriculography and are particularly useful in the acute phase of MI and objectify ventricular disorders and their possible reversibility related to medical or surgical treatment.

References

1 Adam WE, Tarkowska A, Bitter F, Stauch M, Geffers H (1979) Equilibrium gated radionuclide ventriculography. Cardiovasc Radiol 2:161

2 Brochier M, Planiol Th, Itti R, Pellois A (1978) Apport des techniques isotopiques dans le bilan des sujets atteints d'insuffisance coronarienne chronique. Coeur 9: 313

3 Brochier M, Planiol T, Itti R, Pellois A (1978) Interet de la gamma cineangiographie pour l'etude de la fonction ventriculaire gauche a la phase aigue de l'infarctus du myocarde. Ann Cardiol Angeiol (Paris) 27:447
4 Bussman WD, Mayer V, Kober G, Kaltenbach M (1979) Ventricular function at rest, during leg raising and physical exercise before and after aortocoronary bypass surgery. Am J Cardiol 43:488
5 Cohen MV, Downey JM, Sonnenblick EH, Kirke S (1973) The effects of nitroglycerin on coronary collaterals and myocardial contractility. J Clin Invest 52:2836
6 Epstein SE (1973) Hypotension, T.N.G., and acute myocardial infarction. Circulation 47:217
7 Horwitz LD, Herman MV, Gorlin R (1972) Clinical responses to T.N.G. as a diagnosis test for coronary artery disease. Am J Cardiol 29:149
8 Itti R, Planiol T, Pellois A, Brochier M (1979) Etude regionale de la fonction ventriculaire gauche par gamma-cinecardiographie. Medica 65:402
9 Planiol Th, Brochier M, Itti R, Morand Ph, Raynaud Ph, Pellois A (1978) Etude compare et ventriculographie. Arch Mal Coeur 71:132
10 Richtie JL, Sorensen SG, Kennedy JW, Hamilton GW (1979) Radionuclide angiography: non invasive assessment of hemodynamic changes after administration of nitroglycerin. Am J Cardiol 43:278
11 Shad N, Nickel O (1979) Assessment of ventricular function by first-pass angiocardiography. Cardiovasc Radiol 24:149

Thallium Scintigraphy*

H. Schicha, P. Rentrop, K.R. Karsch, L. Facorro, H. Blanke,
H. Kreuzer, and D. Emrich

It was thallium-201 which allowed the application of myocardial scintigraphy in clinical practice [1, 12, 13]. On the one hand, it was expected to supplement coronary angiography as to the microcirculation. On the other hand it was hoped that myocardial scintigraphy could be used as a screening procedure to select patients for invasive investigations. As with all newly introduced methods, it is now important to show its limitations in addition to its usefullnes. These limitations must be known to avoid discrediting of the method due to incorrect indications and to allow critical interpretation of the results.

Like potassium, thallium-201 is concentrated in viable myocardium. Therefore, decreased thallium uptake is seen after transmural myocardial infarction. Stress ischemia reduces thallium uptake after exercise with normalization at rest. Reading of scintigrams is usually performed qualitatively. Quantitative evaluation of digitized data using a computer is more complicated, but significantly increases reproducibility as well as sensitivity [8, 21]. We use a quantitative method for evaluation (Table 1). Stress and redistribution scintigrams are each taken in four views. Data are digitized with a 128 matrix [16], smoothed, normalized, and corrected for background. Then the relative activity distribution is calculated using a fourteen-half-segment model. For quantification of the extent and the degree of a reduced thallium uptake, a thallium score was developed. The method was published in detail [11, 28].

Table 2 shows the sensitivity of thallium scintigraphy for coronary artery disease in a total of 978 patients reported by 17 authors with rather large differences. So, sensitivity at rest ranged between 35% and 65% with a mean value of 50%. Sensitivity after exercise was significantly higher at 62%–98%, 78% being the average.

These differing results might be due to several factors: (1) differences in methodology; (2) differences in observer performance; (3) differences as to specificity, which ranged between 69% and 95%, and/or (4) differences in the composition of the patients investigated.

We would like to point out such differences using our own data. The lower line of Table 2 shows the sensitivity for coronary artery disease in 60 patients using our quantitative method. The overall sensitivity was relatively high; i.e., 70% at rest and 92% after maximum exercise [29].

Twenty normal individuals and 60 patients with coronary artery disease were examined (Table 3). Thirty four patients had previous myocardial infarction. Thirteen patients had one-vessel disease, fourteen had two-vessel disease, and thirty three patients had three-vessel disease. One hundred and forty major vessels were stenosed by

* Supported by SFB 89, Cardiology Göttingen

Table 1. Scintigraphic technique

^{201}Tl:	2 mCi
Camera:	LEM, Searle
Collimator:	Low-energy convergence
Discrimination:	60–89 KeV
Views:	AP, LAO–45°, LAO–60°, LL
Time:	3–6 min for each image

Exercise

Bicycle ergometry in supine position
Maximum exercise limited by severe angina, maximal heart rate, fatigue.
Mean exercise: CAD patients 75 W, normals 143 W.
Injection at peak exercise
Continuation of exercise for 1–3 min
Beginning of exercise scintigraphy 5–6 min after injection
Beginning of rest scintigraphy 2 h after injection

Evaluation

Visualization

Analogue scintigrams (36-mm film)
Digitized scintigrams (color display)

Quantification

Computer:	General data
Matrix:	128 x 128
	Normalization
	Smoothing
	Background substraction
	14-half-segment model

Receiver Operator Characteristic Curves (ROC analysis)

Assessment of sensitivities at a specificity of 90%

at least 50%, of which 44 perfused areas with previous infarction. Receiver operator characteristic curves were used for analysis [17, 18]. All data are calculated at a specificity of 90%.

Two main questions were examined: (1) How sensitive is thallium scintigraphy for detection of coronary artery disease?; and (2) How sensitive is thallium scintigraphy for detection of stenosed vessel, that is, for determination of the extent of the disease?

Figure 1 shows that sensitivity of thallium scintigraphy depended heavily on whether there has been previous infarction. The rest values are shown as open columns, the exercise values as shaded columns. One can see on the left that sensitivity for coronary artery disease in patients with infarction was 88% at rest and 97% after exercise. However, in patients without infarction, sensitivity at rest was significantly lower (46%) and rose after exercise to 85%. On the right the myocardial areas that are perfused by stenosed vessels are shown. For areas with previous infarction, sensitivity at

Table 2. Sensitivity of Thallium scintigraphy for CAD

Reference		n	Rest	Exercise	Rest/exercise
Bailey et al.	[2]	63	49%	62%	75%
Blood et al.	[3]	62	56%	90%	93%
Bodenheimer et al.	[4]	49	–	81%	–
Botvinick et al.	[5]	65	–	85%	–
Buell et al.	[6]	38	62%	–	–
Burguet et al.	[7]	24	44%	–	–
Hamilton et al.	[9]	107	35%	66%	77%
Lenaers et al.	[14]	70	–	–	95%
Loesse et al.	[15]	130	–	98%	–
McLaughlin et al.	[19]	26	–	75%	–
McKillop et al.	[20]	47	–	91%	–
Pabst et al.	[22]	26	–	–	77%
Pachinger et al.	[23]	53	65%	–	–
Ritchie et al.	[26]	76	38%	66%	76%
Turner et al.	[30a]	34	–	68%	–
Verani et al.	[31, 32]	48	–	–	79%
Range			35%–65%	62%–98%	75%–95%
Mean		918	50%	78%	82%
Schicha et al.	[28, 29]	60	70%	92%	94%

Table 3. Patient population and methodology

	Total	Normals	CAD with-out MI	CAD with MI
Number of patients	80	20	26	34
Age (years) mean		41	53	53
One-vessel disease	13	0	8	5
Two-vessel disease	14	0	6	8
Three-vessel disease	33	0	12	21

rest was 86% and after exercise 93%. For areas without infarction sensitivity was significantly lower at rest (26%) and rose even after maximum exercise to only 67%.

Figure 2 shows the dependency of the sensitivity of thallium scintigraphy on the number of diseased vessels. The left part of the figure points out that in patients without infarction, sensitivity for coronary artery disease was high in one-vessel and two-vessel disease, being 75% and 71% at rest and 88% and 100% after exercise. However, in three-vessel disease sensitivity was significantly lower – only 23% at rest and 69% after exercise. The right side of Fig. 2 shows the sensitivity for areas without infarction. In one-vessel disease sensitivity at rest was 50% and after exercise 88%. In two-vessel disease sensitivity was lower, being 29% at rest and 71% after exercise. A further loss of sensitivity occurred in three-vessel disease being only 24% at rest and 56% after exercise. These data clearly demonstrate a reduced sensitivity for detection of coronary

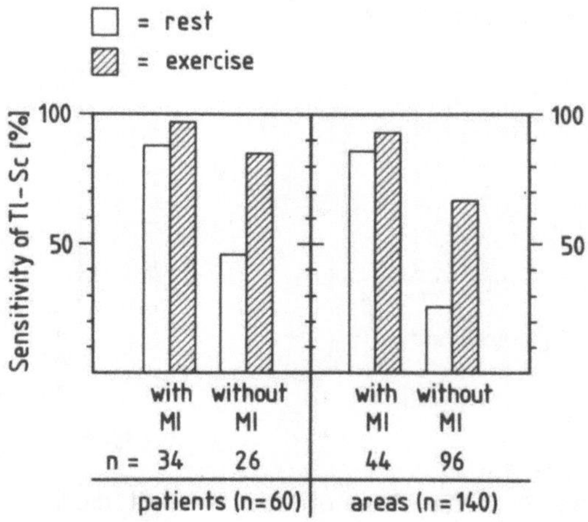

Fig. 1. Sensitivity of thallium scintigraphy (*Tl Sc.*) for patients and for areas with and without previous myocardial infarction (*MI*)

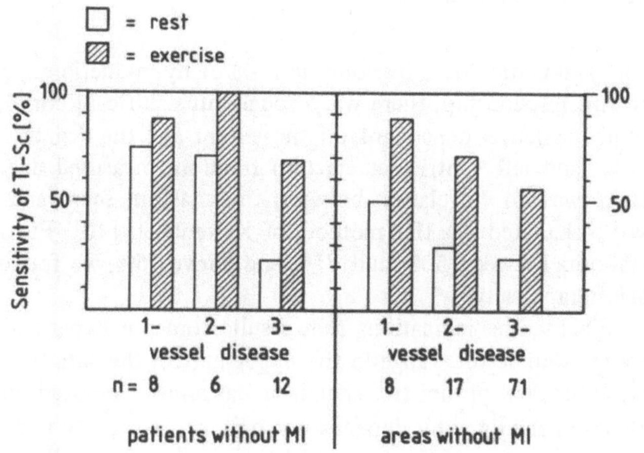

Fig. 2. Sensitivity of thallium scintigraphy (*Tl Sc.*) in relation to the number of stenosed vessels

artery disease as well as for the estimation of its extent in patients with multiple-vessel disease without infarction.

There may be two reasons for this low sensitivity: Either the stenoses might be hemodynamically insignificant, or the sensitivity of thallium scintigraphy is not sufficient in this respect. Several results support the suggestion of insufficient sensitivity.

In 20 selected patients biplane cineventriculography was evaluated during maximum exercise angina (Fig. 3) [24]. Wall motion abnormalities were observed in more than 90% of areas without infarction, which were perfused by vessels with stenoses of 50% and more. However, a reduced thallium uptake was present in only 66% of them. Considering wall motion abnormalities, measured angiographically at rest and, in part, during maximum exercise, we found a reduced thallium uptake in 86% of akinetic

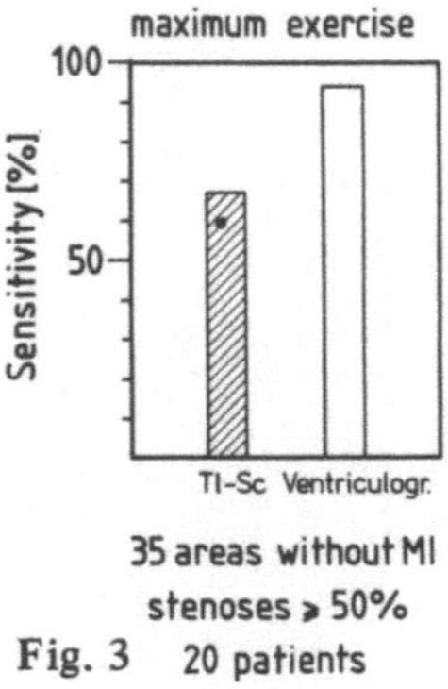

Fig. 3

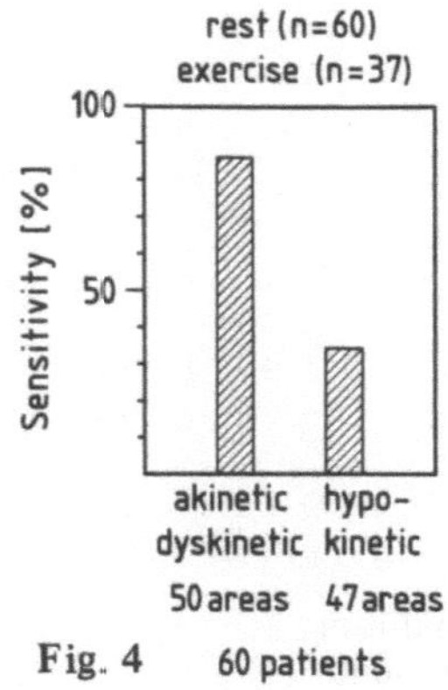

Fig. 4

Fig. 3. Comparison of exercise wall motion abnormalities (*ventriculography* with thallium scintigraphy; *Tl Sc.*)

Fig. 4. Sensitivity of thallium scintigraphy (*Tl Sc.*) for areas with various degrees of wall motion abnormalities

and dyskinetic areas, but only in 34% of hypokinetic regions (Fig. 4). Corresponding to this relationship, there was a rough but significant correlation between the thallium score, which is dependent on the extent and the degree of reduced thallium uptake [11], and left ventricular ejection fraction, measured angiographically (Fig. 5). But there was no correlation between the thallium score and the coronary score, which was calculated by the method of Kaltenbach [10]. Furthermore, after subdividing stenoses between 50% and 75% and above 75%, we found no significant differences scintigraphically.

Finally, the indications that result from our experiences should be discussed. Although our results range in the upper part of the data from the literature, our conclusions are less optimistic. Hamilton has already pointed out that the clinical value of thallium scintigraphy depends not only on sensitivity and specificity, but also on the predictive value of the individual test result. The predictive value depends on the prevalence of the disease in the study population [9].

Table 4 shows the predictive values of either a negative or a positive thallium scintigram, which is dependent on the prevalence of coronary artery disease. With a prevalence of 10%, i.e., in screening, the normal thallium scintigram has a high predictive value of 98%. The positive scintigram, however, has only a low predictive value of 49%. That means that half of the patients with a pathologic scintigram in a population with 10% prevalence do not have coronary artery disease. Such results would be accepted in screening, if the test were simple and inexpensive and could be performed easily. This, however, is not true for thallium scintigraphy.

In the case of typical angina and a high prevalence of, for instance, 90%, the predictive value of a positive scintigram is 99%. However, the negative test result has a predictive value of only 40%. Therefore, when using thallium scintigraphy, it is not acceptable to exclude coronary artery disease and to omit the invasive investigation in patients with typical angina.

Considering a medium prevalence of 50%, as in patients with atypical angina or in asymptomatic patients with a pathologic ECG, thallium scintigraphy has a high pre-

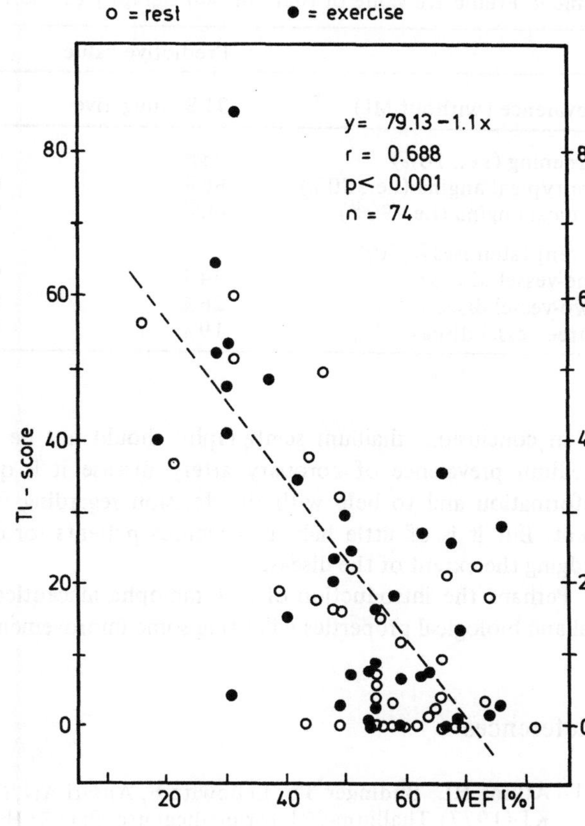

Fig. 5. Correlation between the thallium score and the LVEF, estimated angiographically

dictive value of approximately 85% –90% in proving and excluding coronary artery disease. In our opinion only this is an indication for thallium scintigraphy, to either bring the patient to invasive investigation or to avoid it.

The predictive value of thallium scintigraphy in determining the hemodynamic significance of a stenosed vessel in an area without previous infarction is shown in the lower part of Table 4, assuming a hemodynamic significance with 90% prevalence. While the positive test result has a high predictive value of 98%–99%, the predictive value of a normal thallium uptake in a myocardial area in one-vessel disease is 44%, in two-vessel disease 26%, and in three-vessel disease 19%. These values cannot be accepted for clinical use.

Therefore, thallium scintigraphy is not useful in estimating the extent of coronary artery disease. This is in agreement with the results of McKillop [20]. Thallium scintigraphy also appears not to be useful in recognizing or excluding a hemodynamic significance in borderline stenoses, i.e., between 50%–75%. Therefore, from our point of view, it is problematic to make the indication of a bypass operation dependent on the results of thallium scintigraphy. Also still open to discussion is whether thallium scintigraphy is useful in evaluating the function of aortocoronary bypasses postoperatively [25, 27, 30, 31].

Table 4. Predictive value of thallium scintigraphy (Tl Sc.)

	Predictive value	
Prevalence (without MI)	Tl Sc. negative	Tl Sc. positive
Screening (i.e., 10%)	98%	49%
Nontypical angina (i.e., 50%)	86%	89%
Typical angina (i.e., 90%)	40%	99%
Extent (stenoses ⩾ 50%)		
One-vessel disease	44%	99%
Two-vessel disease	26%	98%
Three-vessel disease	19%	98%

In conclusion, thallium scintigraphy should not be overrated. In patients with a medium prevalence of coronary artery disease it is quite useful to give additional information and to help with the decision regarding further examination of the patient. But it is of little help in screening patients for coronary artery disease and in judging the extent of the disease.

Perhaps the introduction of new radiopharmaceuticals with more favorable physical and biological properties will bring some improvement in this direction.

References

1 Atkins HL, Budinger TF, Lebowitz E, Ansari AN, Greene MW, Fairchild RG, Ellis KJ (1977) Thallium-201 for medical use. Part 3: Human distribution and physical imaging properties. J Nucl Med 18:133
2 Bailey IK, Griffith LSC, Rouleau J, Strauss HW, Pitt B (1977) Thallium-201 myocardial perfusion imaging at rest and during exercise. Circulation 55:79
3 Blood DK, McCarthy DM, Sciacca RR, Cannon PJ (1978) Comparison of single-dose and double-dose-thallium-201 myocardial perfusion scintigraphy for detection of coronary artery disease and prior myocardial infarction. Circulation 58:777
4 Bodenheimer MM, Banka VS, Fouche CM, Helfant RH (1978) Comparative sensitivity of the exercise electrocardiogram, thallium imaging and stress radionuclide angiography to detect the presence and severity of coronary disease. Circulation 57/58 (Suppl II):139
5 Botvinick EH, Taradash MR, Shames DM, Parmley WW (1978) Thallium-201 myocardial perfusion scintigraphy for the clinical clarification of normal, abnormal and equivocal electrocardiographic stress tests. Am J Cardiol 41:43
6 Büll U, Niendorf HP, Strauer BE, Hast B (1976) Evaluation of myocardial function with the 201 Thallium scintimetry in various diseases of heart. Eur J Nucl Med 1:125
7 Burquet W, Beequevort P, Dwelshauvers J, Lenears A, Merchie G (1976) La scintigraphy du myocarde au Tl-201 dans la maladie coronarienne. In: Höfer S (ed) Radioaktive Isotope in Klinik und Forschung, Vol 12. Egermann, Vienna, p 457
8 Emrich D, Rentrop P, Facorro L, Karsch R, Schicha H, Carstens B, Kreuzer H (1978) Limitations of thallium-201 scintigraphy for evaluation of chronic ischemic heart disease. 2nd Int Congr World Fed Nucl Med Biol, Washington, Sept 1978
9 Hamilton GW, Trobaugh GB, Ritchie JL, Gould KL, De Rouen TA, Williams DL (1978) Myocardial imaging with thallium-201: An analyses of clinical usefullness based on Bayes theorem. Semin Nucl Med 8:358

10 Kaltenbach M (1975) Quantitative Bewertung koronarangiographischer Befunde mit Hilfe eines Punktesystems (Score) Z Kardiol 64:597
11 Karsch KR, Schicha H, Rentrop P, Blanke H, Kreuzer H, Emrich D (to be published) Quantitative Thallium-201 Szintigraphie in der Diagnostik von Ausmaß und Ausdehnung der koronaren Herzerkrankung. Vergleich eines Tl-Scores mit invasiven und nichtinvasiven Daten. Z Kardiol
12 Kawana M, Krizek H, Porter J, Lathrop D, Charleston D, Harper PV (1970) Use of Tl-199 as a potassium analog in scanning (Abstract). J Nucl Med 11:333
13 Lebowitz E, Greene MW, Fairchild F, Bradley-Moore PR, Atkins HL, Ansari AN, Richards P, Belgrave E (1975) Thallium-201 for medical use. J Nucl Med 16:151
14 Lenaers A, Block P, van Thiel E, Lebedelle M, Bequevort P, Erbsman F, Ermans AM (1977) Segmental analysis of Tl-201 stress myocardial scintigraphy. J Nucl Med 18:509
15 Lösse B, Krönert H, Rafflenbeul D, Feinendegen LE, Loogen F (1979) Empfindlichkeit und Treffsicherheit der Thallium-201-Myokardszintigraphie bei der Diagnostik der koronaren Herzkrankheit und von Myokardschäden anderer Ursache. Z Kardiol 68:429
16 Luig H, Lahne R, Domowitz S (1977) Ein Datensystem für kardiologische Untersuchungen mit einer Gamma-Kamera. In: Lorenz WJ (ed) Medizinische Physik, Vol II. Berlin, p 99
17 Lusted LB (1968) Introduction to medical decision making. Springfield
18 Lusted LB (1978) General problems in medical decision making with comments on ROC analyses. Semin Nucl Med 8:299
19 McLaughlin PR, Martin RP, Doherty P, Daspit S, Goris M, Haskell W, Lewis St, Kriss JP, Harrison D (1977) Reproducibility of thallium-201 myocardial imaging. Circulation 55:497
20 McKillop JH, Murray RG, Turner JG, Bessent RG, Lorimer AR, Greig WG (1979) Can the extent of coronary artery disease be predicted from thallium-201 myocardial images? J Nucl Med 20:715
21 Meade RC, Bamrah VS, Horgan JD, Ruetz PP, Kronenwetter C, Yeh EL (1978) Quantitative methods in the evaluation of thallium-201 myocardial perfusion images. J Nucl Med 19:1175
22 Pabst HW, Hör G, Lichte H, Sebening H, Kriegel H (1976) Experience with thallium-201 in detection of myocardial infarction. Eur J Nucl Med 1:19
23 Pachinger O, Probst P, Orgis E, Kaindl E (1977) Quantitative 201-Thallium-Myokardszintigraphie bei koronarer Herzkrankheit. Herz-Kreisl 9:310
24 Rentrop P, Karsch KR, Schichta H (to be published) Limitations of Tl-201 exercise scintigraphy in coronary artery disease. A correlation with coronary angiography and exercise ventriculography. Internat Cardiovasc Congr II, Febr 1979. Scottsdale
25 Ritchie JL, Narahara KA, Trobaugh GB, Williams DL, Hamilton GW (1977) Thallium-201 myocardial imaging before and after coronary revascularization: assessment of regional myocardial blood flow and graft patency. Circulation 56: 830
26 Ritchie JL, Trobaugh B, Hamilton GW, Gould KL, Naraharam KA, Murray JA (1977) Myocardial imaging with thallium-201 at rest and during exercise: Comparison with coronary arteriography and resting and stress electrocardiography. Circulation 56:66
27 Robinson PS, Williams BT, Webb-Peploe MM, Crowther A, Coltart DJ (1979) Thallium-201 myocardial imaging in assessment of results of artocoronary bypass surgery. Br Heart J 42:455
28 Schicha H, Facorro L, Rentrop P, Karsch R, Blanke H, Luig B, Carstens B, Domowitz S, Kreuzer H, Emrich D (1979) Quantitative Belastungs-Szintigraphie des Myokards mit 201-Tl-Methodik und Normalverhalten. Nucl Med 6:266
29 Schicha H, Rentrop P, Facorro L, Karsch KR, Blanke H, Kreuzer H, Emrich D (1980) Ergebnisse der quantitativen Myokardszintigraphie mit Thallium-201 in

Ruhe und unter maximaler Belastung – Kritische Analyse des prädiktiven Wertes und der klinischen Anwendung. Z Kardiol 69:31

30 Schicha H, Blanke H, Rentrop P, Karsch KR, Kreuzer H, Emrich D (to be published) Myokardszintigraphie mit Thallium-201 zur Feststellung der Funktionsfähigkeit aortokoronarer Bypasse mit Mehrfach-KHK und Mehrfach-Bypassen. Z Kardiol

30a Turner DA, Battle WE, Deshmukh H, Colandrea MA, Suycer GJ, Fordham EW, Messer JV (1978) The predictive value of myocardial perfusion scintigraphy after stress in patients without previous myocardial infarction. J Nucl Med 19: 249

31 Verani MS, Marcus ML, Spoto G, Rossi NP, Ehrhardt JC, Razzak MA (1978) Thallium-201 myocardial perfusion scintigrams in the evaluation of aorto-coronary saphenous bypass surgery. J Nucl Med 19:765

32 Verani MS, Marcus ML, Razzak MA, Ehrhardt JC (1978) Sensitivity and specificity of thallium-201 perfusion scintigrams under exercise in the diagnostic of coronary artery disease. J Nucl Med 19:773

Myocardial Scintigraphy with Free Fatty Acids and Glucose

K. Vyska, C. Freundlieb, A. Höck, L.E. Feinendegen, G. Kloster,
H.J. Machulla, and G. Stöcklin

For objective evaluation of myocardial ischemia and for characterization of cryptogenic cardiomyopathy, quantitative information about myocardial metabolism is necesary [24, 31]. For external monitoring of myocardial metabolism in vivo, radiopharmaceuticals are needed which are directly incorporated into the metabolic pathway in the myocardium. Therefore, much effort was invested in developing suitable labeling procedures for metabolic substrates [5, 8, 12, 14, 18, 19, 20, 22, 27].

In the Institutes of Medicine and of Nuclear Chemistry of the Nuclear Research Center in Jülich we first concentrated on the development of radioactively labeled free fatty acids (RLFFA) [6, 15, 28]. These seem to be particularly useful for the detection of metabolic alterations associated with ischemia, since free fatty acids are known to be the main physiologic substrate for myocardial energy production [1, 10, 16, 23], their enzymatic breakdown requires aerobic conditions [4, 10], and their myocardial extraction is drastically reduced under conditions of hypoxia and normal perfusion [10, 30, 31].

In order to find the most suitable isotope and the optimal labeling position for different fatty acids we first labeled a variety of them in ω- and a-position with bromine-77, fluorine-18, chlorine-34m, iodine-123, and carbon-11 (see Fig. 1) and injected them into mice [15]. The highest uptake was found for heptadecanoic acid labeled in ω-position with iodine-123 (see Fig. 2). It was equal to that observed for ^{11}C-palmitic acid. Poorer results were obtained with ω-cloro- and ω-bromofatty acids and with a-halofatty acids. The smaller uptake of ω-chloro- and ω-bromofatty acids can be explained by a stronger binding to proteins, while the poor uptake of the a-halofatty acids seems to be due to steric and inductive effects that influence esterification of fatty acids coenzyme A (CoA) and carnitine and thereby inhibit their passage through the mitochondrial membrane.

These results led us to conclude that for carrying out metabolic studies the most suitable radiopharmaceuticals are ^{11}C-palmitic acid and ω- ^{123}I-heptadecanoic acid.

Since ^{11}C is a posinotron emitter, ^{11}C-palmatic acid can be effectively used only in conjunction with positron-emission computer-assisted tomography.

Due to the almost pure 155 keV gamma radiation of ^{123}I, ω- ^{123}I-heptadecanoic acid (IHA) can be detected with any commercially available γ-camera. Since the atomic diameter of iodine ($\sim$ 2 Å) is very similar to the diameter of the methyl group (see Fig. 3), IHA may be considered to be the steric analogue of stearic acid.

The images obtained with IHA are of high quality [7, 28]. Figure 4 shows a typical background-corrected [7] normal myocardial image obtained in anterior projection at rest. The myocardium is clearly delineated from all surrounding tissues. Only the left ventricle is visualized whereas the right ventricle cannot usually be recognized

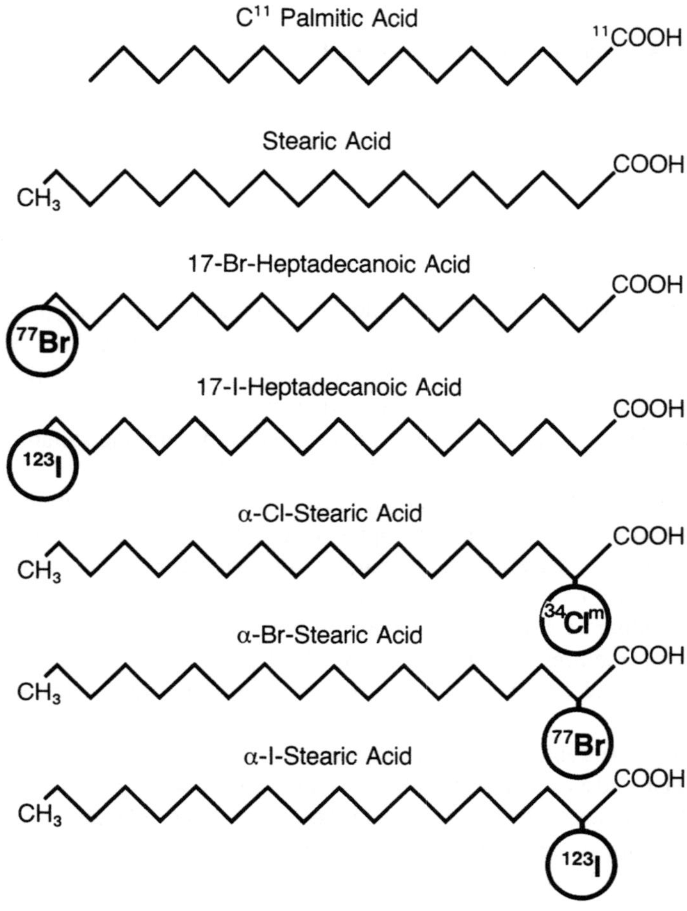

Fig. 1. Summary of radioactively labeled fatty acids which were used in animal described in this paper

because of its small myocardial muscle mass. The acitivity distribution in the left myocardium is seen to be homogeneous.

The images obtained in 35 patients suffering from coronary artery disease and nine patients with old myocardial infarction [7, 9, 28] demonstrated that in IHA scintigrams infarcted areas as well as ischemic regions can be easily recognized as areas with reduced activity accumulation (see Fig. 5). When compared to ^{201}TI scintigraphy these defects were found to be more pronounced and usually already detectable at rest. During moderate exercise (at about 40–50 W) the accumulation defects in ischemic regions were accentuated [9, 28].

Figure 6 shows the myocardial image of a patient with coronary artery disease, taken in LAO 45° projection at rest. The arteriogram, shown on the right, demonstrates the 50% and 30% narrowing of the right coronary artery. Also in this case the activity accumulation defect was registered even at rest, i.e., with a high probability under conditions of normal perfusion in the diseased region.

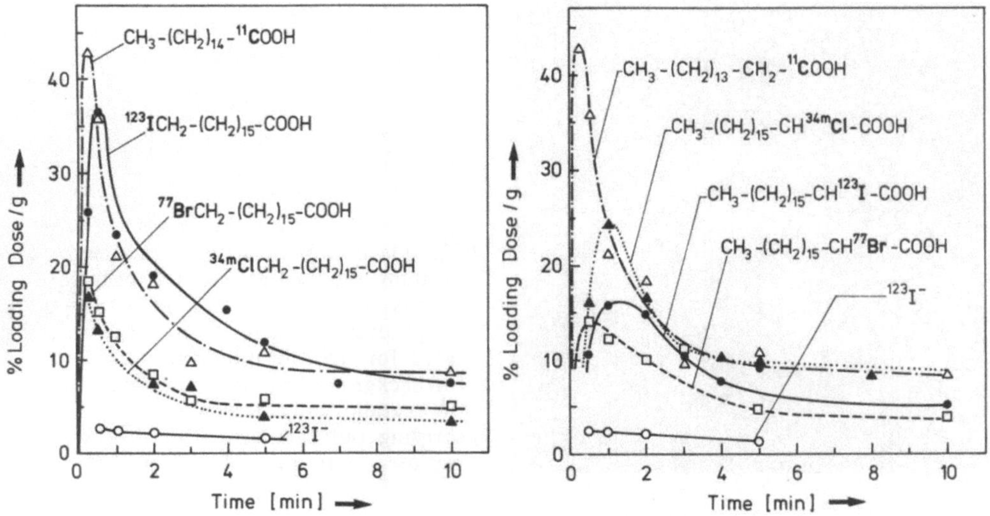

Fig. 2a, b. The time course of radioactivity in mouse heart muscle after intravenous (i.v.) injection of: **a** 17-^{34m}Cl-, 17-^{77}Br-, 17-^{123}I-heptadecanoic acid, [1-^{11}C] plamitic acid, and ionic ^{123}I; **b** α-^{34m}Cl, α-^{77}Br-, α-^{123}I-stearic acid [1-^{11}C] palmitic acid, and ionic ^{123}I; (200 μl 6% HSA solution containing 100 nCi). Average deviations are within ± 22% of indicated values

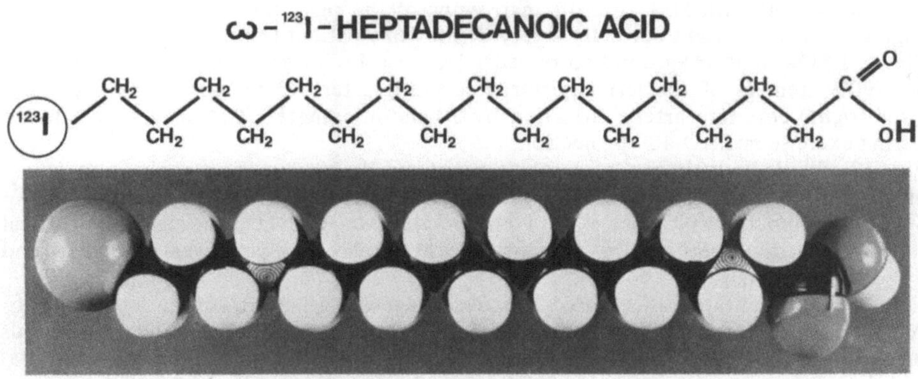

Fig. 3. Structural model of ω-^{123}I-heptadecanoic acid

Taking these results into account it must be concluded that the regional accumulation of IHA in the myocardium not only reflects local perfusion but also depends on the regional ability of the myocardium to extract the supplied substrate.

Under conditions of ischemia not only the fatty acid supply and its extraction but also its catabolism are expected to be changed.

Information about fatty acid catabolism can be obtained by analyzing IHA elimination rates [7, 9, 28]. The elimination of IHA from normal myocardium follows a mono-

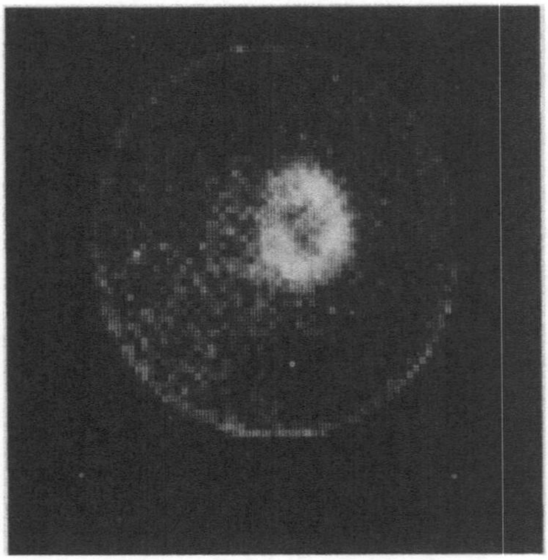

Fig. 4. Anterior image of normal myocardium obtained at 7 min after intravenous injection of 2.0 mCi ω-^{123}I-heptadecanoic acid. This image was gated for diastole only and corrected for background activity resulting from the catabolically released ^{123}I. For carrying out this correction ^{123}I-NaI was used as an internal standard [7]

Fig. 5. Anterior IHA myocardial images (gated and background corrected) from normal person (*left*), patient with an apical infarction (9 years old) (*middle*), and patient with CAD (*right*)

Fig. 6. LAO 60° IHA myocardial image (gated and background corrected) from a 49-year-old patient with 50% and 30% narrowing of the right coronary artery (*left*) and angiography of the right coronary artery of the same patient (*right*)

Fig. 9. ECG-gated background-corrected IHA diastolic images of a patient with proximal 90% stenosis of the left anterior descending artery, detected before (*left*) and after (*right*) coronary artery dilatation by a balloon catheter. The images were taken during exercise in LAO 40° projection

Fig. 13. Whole-body image of a rabbit registered 4–10 min after application of 1.5 mCi 3-^{11}C-methyl-D-glucose (MG), by means of a large field of view γ-camera (LFOV Searle), equipped with a special (511 keV) collimator (*left*). On the *right*, the vertical slice through the myocardium, demonstrating the relationship between the heart and liver MG accumulation

Fig. 15. Representative ECG-gated diastolic image of the myocardium at the level of A-V valves, obtained by positron-emission, transaxial tomography, after intravenous injection of 2 mCi ^{11}C-methyl glucose in a lightly anesthetized dog. Both ventricles are clearly delineated and imposed with homogeneous distribution of activity in myocardium. The central areas within the horseshoe patterns correspond to the left and right ventricular cavities. The transmission image (*left*), obtained with the use of ^{68}Ge as a positron source, at the same level was used to indicate the location of the heart within the thorax and to obtain attenuation factors prior to intravenous injections of ^{11}C-methyl glucose

Fig. 16. Image obtained with a positron-emission transaxial tomograph, in a subject suffering from arterial fibrillation, with no pulse deficit, after intravenous administration of 1.5 mCi ^{11}C-methyl glucose. The section is viewed from a cephalad-to-caudad orientation, in accordance with conventions in transmission tomography. The collection period was 6 min. As can be seen, the characteristic distribution of MG is circular at the midventricular level, whereas it conforms to a horseshoe-shaped pattern (see Fig. 15) at the level of the A-V valves, where the posterior portion of the heart comprises left atrial rather than ventricular myocardium

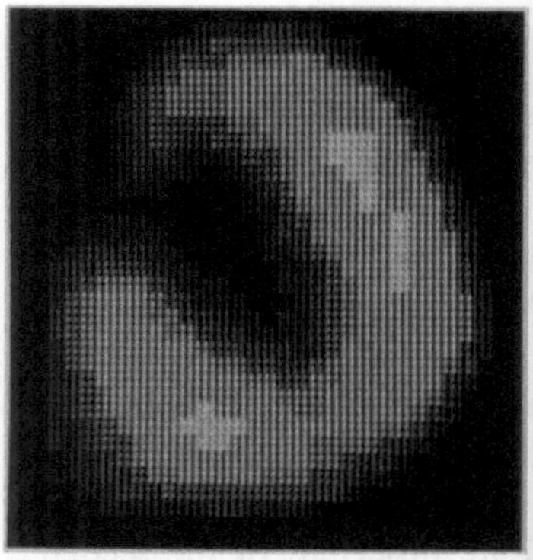

5a Normal myocardium

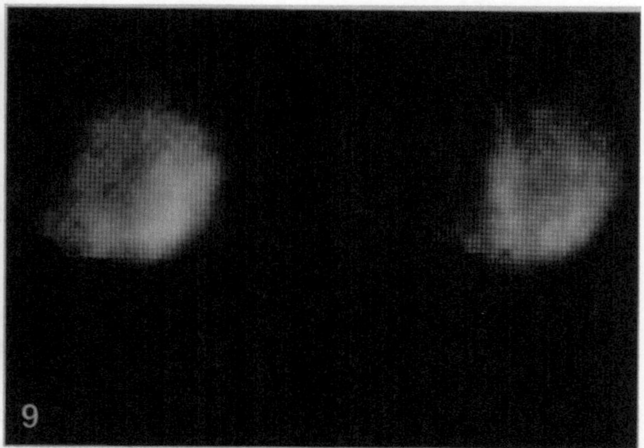

9

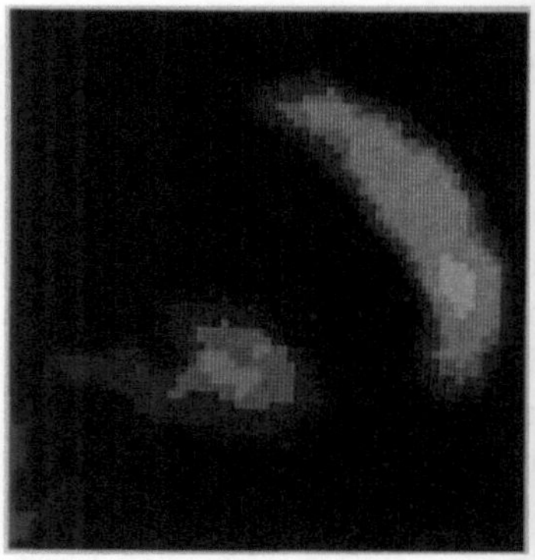

5b Apical infarction

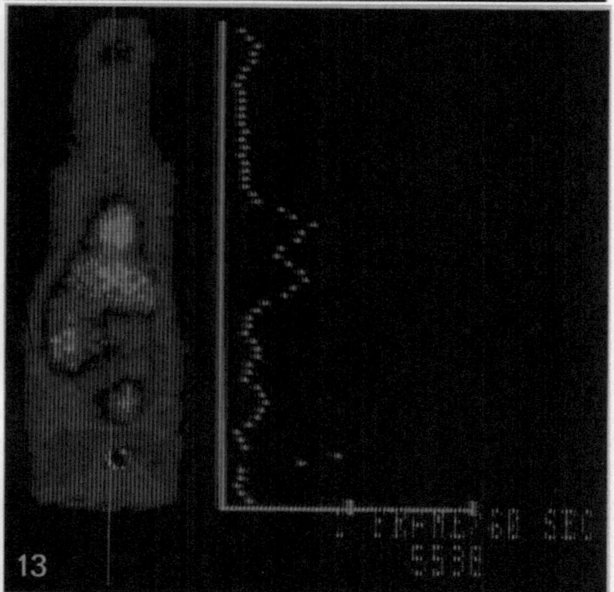

13

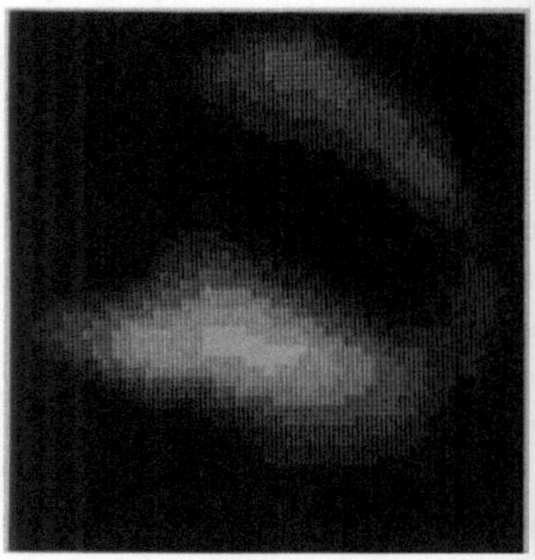

5c Coronary heart disease

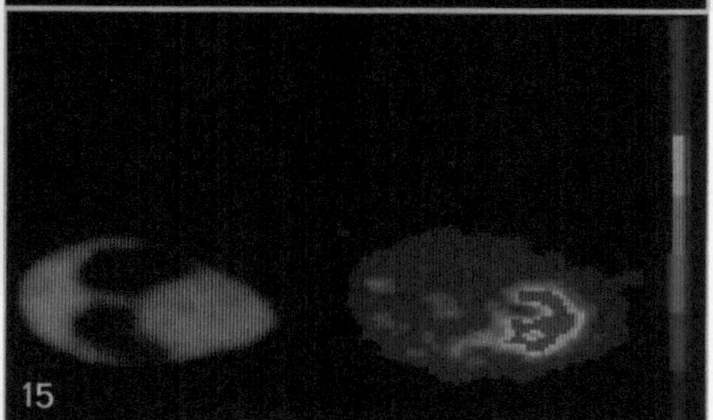

15

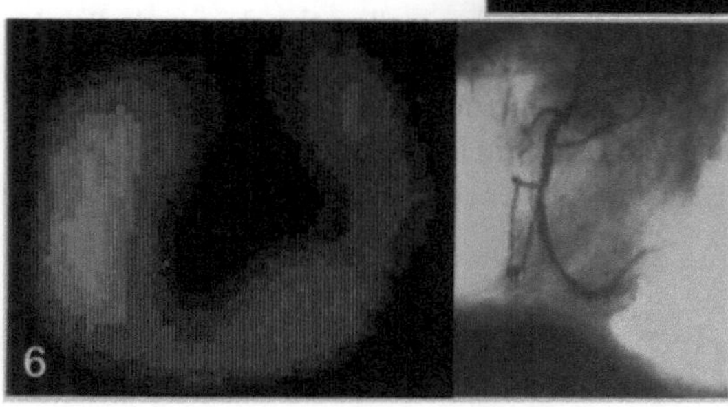

6

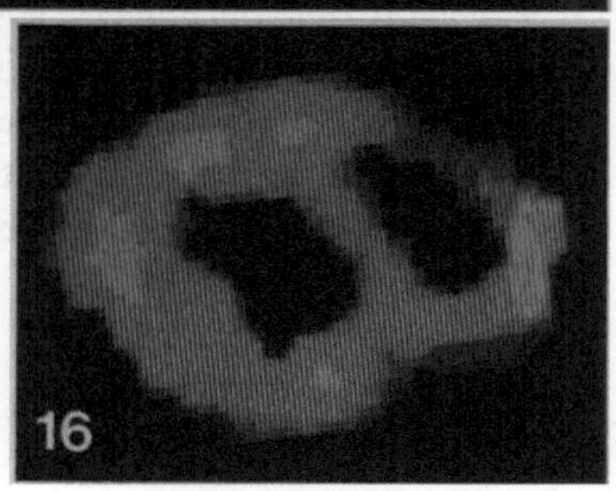

16

exponential function with a half-life of 25 ± 5 min (see Fig. 7). In Fig. 8 the time activity curves obtained in a patient with coronary artery disease (CAD) are demonstrated. As can be seen, the half-time of IHA elimination from the lateral part of the left ventricular wall, where indicator accumulation is diminished, is significantly prolonged. It was found to be 42 min. The half-time of IHA elimination in the septal area was 30 min.

The data obtained so far in 35 patients with coronary artery disease, examined at rest, indicate that these patients can be subdivided into two groups according to the rate of fatty acid elimination. In the first group, in the area of accumulation defects, prolonged half-times of IHA elimination (30–70 min) are observed. In the second group, in areas of accumulation defects, normal or slightly shortened half-times of IHA elimination are detected. These results indicate that in areas of diminished IHA accumulation, a normal as well as pathologically altered fatty acid turnover may exist.

Following the period of exercise the half-times of IHA elimination in areas of accumulation defects became significantly prolonged, whereas in normal areas, no exercise-dependent changes in IHA elimination half-times were observed [7, 9].

Five patients, three of them with normal and two with prolonged IHA elimination in areas of accumulation defect, were examined before and after coronary artery dilatation by balloon catheter [30]. Figure 9 shows (on the left) the IHA myocardial image of a patient with a proximal 90% stenosis of the left anterior descending artery. The image was taken before coronary artery dilatation during exercise in LAO 45° projection. IHA accumulation in the septal area is drastically reduced. After coronary artery dilatation, the accumulation in the septal area became normal, as shown on the right.

Also in two other patients, with normal half-times of IHA elimination in the area of the accumulation defect, the accumulation defect disappeared after coronary artery dilatation.

In order to interpret these observations and to clarify the pharmacokinetics of RLFFA, we carried out separate experiments with mice [3]. In these experiments, the animals were killed at different time intervals after IHA application, the hearts were homogenized and fractionated, and the activity in water and organic phases as well as in tissue residue was determined. The results obtained are summarized in Figs. 10 and 11. As can be seen in Fig. 11, where the results of fractionation of organic phase by means of thin-layer chromatography are demonstrated, IHA appears immediately after intravenous application in fractions comigrating with phospholipids and free fatty acids. After some time delay, it is detected in the fraction comigrating with triglycerides. These results, which closely agree with the data obtained by Stein et al. [25, 26], support the hypothesis that in the myocardial cell a triglyceride pool with a very high turnover exists, which serves as an easily mobilizable fatty acid store. When the myocardial energy consumption is increased, the free fatty acids can be mobilized from this pool as acyl-S-CoA and follow the usual metabolic pathway for fatty acids. It is evident that the changes in such a triglyceride pool as well as the changes in β-oxidation rate, which are known to occur under the conditions of ischemia, must be considered as possible causes for alterations in IHA elimination rates. The data obtained by Idell-Wenger et al. [11] on isolated ischemic hearts, which indicate that the availability of carnitine in the cytosol might be highly reduced under conditions of repeated transient

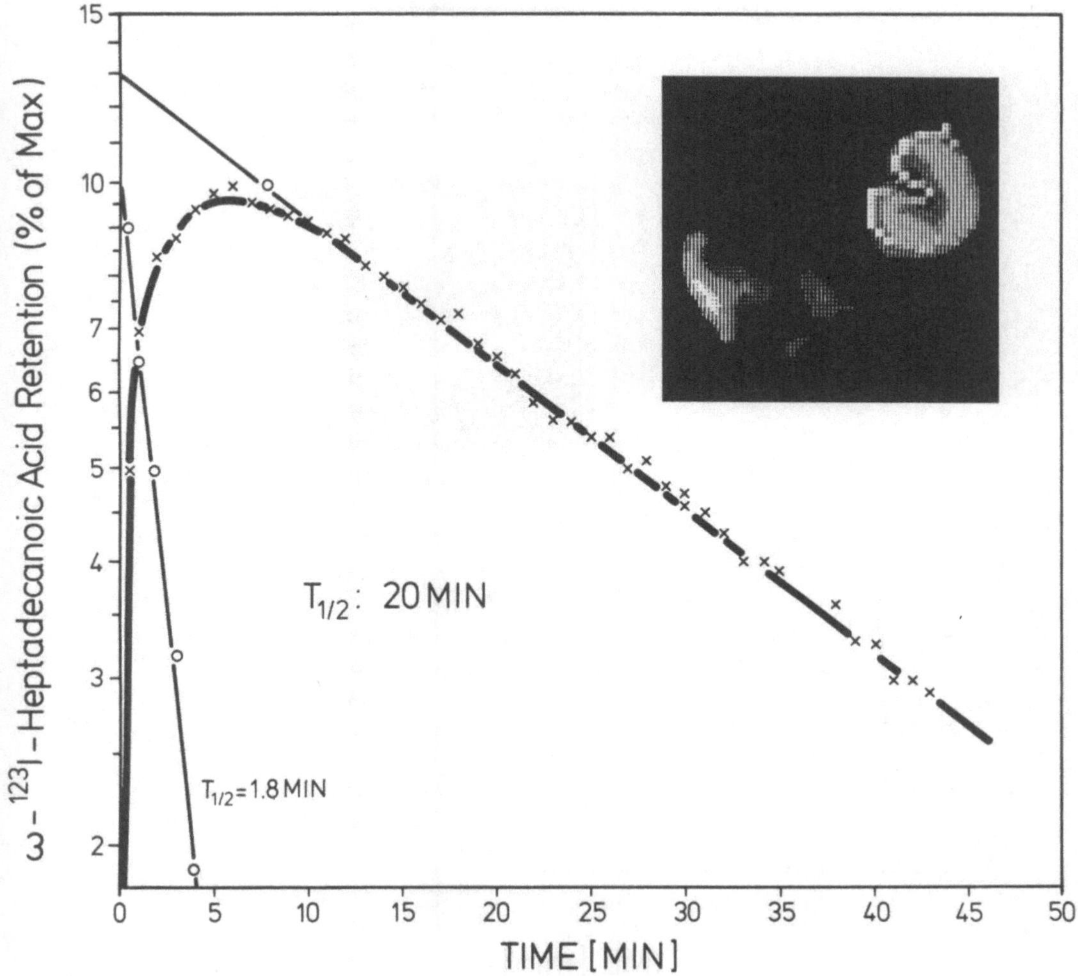

Fig. 7. Background-corrected [7] IHA turnover curve detected over the myocardium in a normal subject

ischemia, demonstrate, moreover, that the ischemia-dependent changes in the carnitine shuttle system may also lead to alterations in IHA elimination rates.

Even if these results do not allow full interpretation of all our observations, they demonstrate that in ischemic myocardium significant alterations in free fatty acid metabolic pathways exist which may be traced by the use of IHA as an indicator. This means that ω-I-heptadecanoic acid represents not only a suitable tracer for the external detection of the regional availability of fatty acids for myocardial energy production but also for detection of the ischemia-dependent alterations of the rate of regional fatty acid utilization. We expect, moreover, that the information obtained by the use of IHA as an indicator might contribute in the future to the quantification of the viability of myocardial tissue exposed to repeated transient ischemic insults.

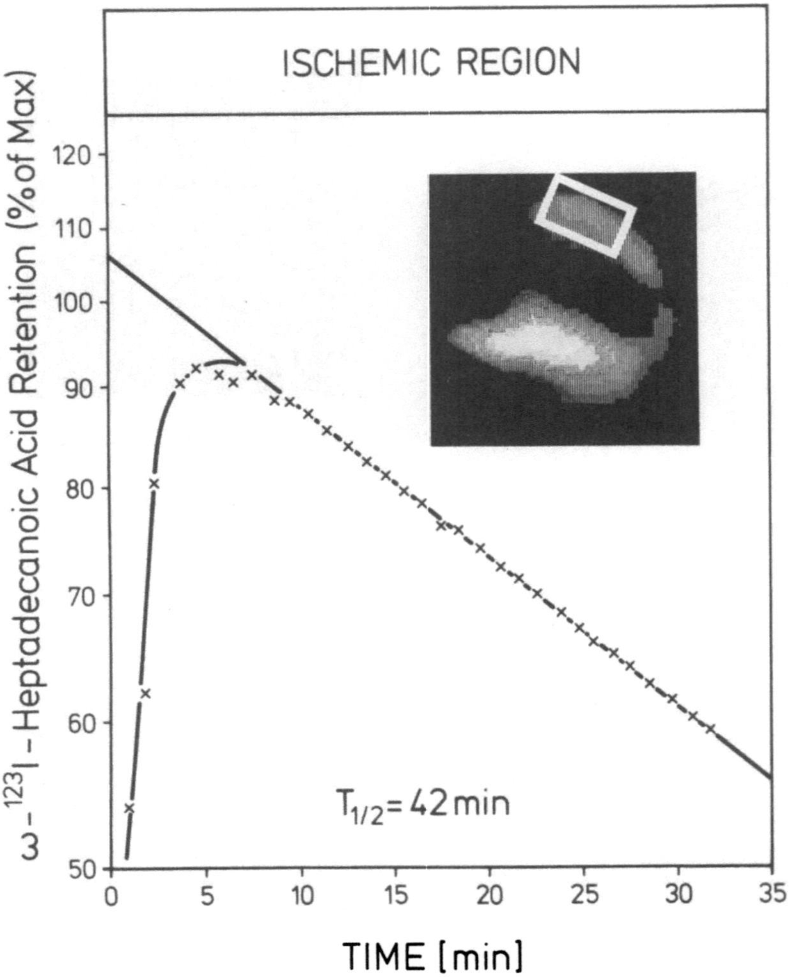

Fig. 8a, b. Background-corrected [7] IHA turnover curves registered over different regions of myocardium in a patient suffering from CAD

In the discussion of cell viability it must, however, be considered that not only the knowledge of fatty acid metabilism but also information on the myocardial cell membrane is necessary.

Since fatty acid passage through the cell membrane is probably only a passive process, IHA cannot be considered as an indicator suitable for external detection of the state and function of the myocardial cell membrane. In order to obtain information about the state of myocardial cell membrane, an indicator is needed which is actively transported across the cell membrane but which is not metabolized.

Based on reports from in vitro studies, radioactively labeled methyl glucose (MG) was chosen as an indicator fulfilling these conditions [2, 17, 21, 29, 32]. Similar to glucose, MG is also transported across the cell membrane by carrier-facilitated, ATP-dependent mechanisms, but it does not enter the glycolytic pathway [21, 32]. The

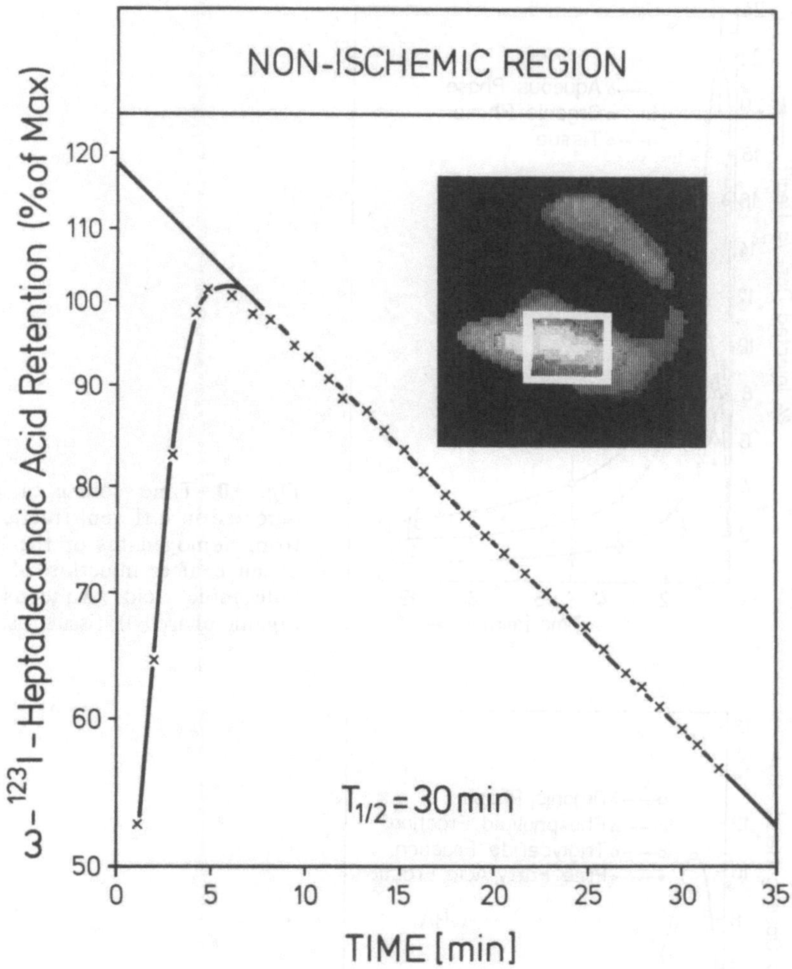

Fig. 8b

transport of MG was found to be stimulated under conditions of acute hypoxia but is drastically reduced under the conditions of anoxia [21].

For in vivo studies MG was labeled with ^{11}C. The ^{11}C-methyl glucose was synthesized by methylation via $^{11}CH_3I$ of potassium salt of diacetone D-glucose (see Fig. 12) [13]. The radioactively labeled MG was first injected intravenously into rabbits and dogs.

In rabbits the whole-body distribution of MG was registered with a γ-camera equipped with a special (511 keV) collimator. As shown in Fig. 13, methyl glucose is preferentially accumulated in the heart, liver, brain, and kidney. The myocardium is clearly delineated from all surrounding tissues. The heart/lung and the heart/liver ratios were found to be 3.3 and 1, respectively. The turnover of MG in the myocardium was rapid with accumulation and elimination half-times of 2 and 5 min, respectively.

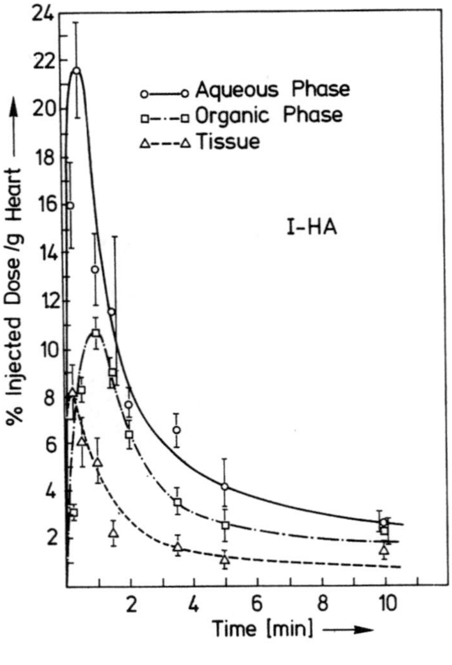

Fig. 10. Time course of radioactivity detected in different fractions extracted from homogenates of the heart muscle of mice after injection of ω-^{131}I-heptadecanoic acid. Aqueous phase (○); organic phase (□); tissue residue (△)

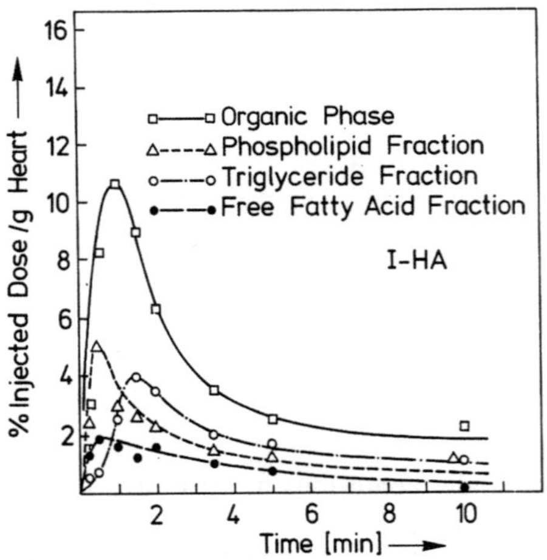

Fig. 11. Time course of radioactivity in various fractions extracted from the heart of mice after injection of ω-^{131}I-heptadecanoic acid. Average deviations are within ± 25% of indicated values

The activity distribution in dog experiments was registered by means of an emission computer-assisted tomograph (see Fig. 14). Figure 15 shows, on the right, a typical image of the normal dog heart in diastole at the level of A-V valves, detected 5 min after application of 2 mCi ^{11}C-methyl glucose. The scintigram demonstrates homogeneous activity distribution in both left and right myocardium. The transmission image registered at the same level is shown on the left.

A typical tomographic image of the human myocardium is seen in Fig. 16. The patient suffers from arterial hypertension well controlled by therapy but with atrial

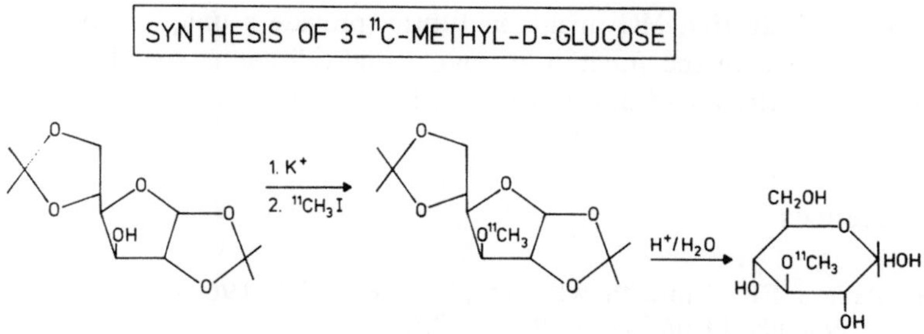

Fig. 12. Schematic representation of the synthesis of 3-^{11}C-methyl-D-glucose

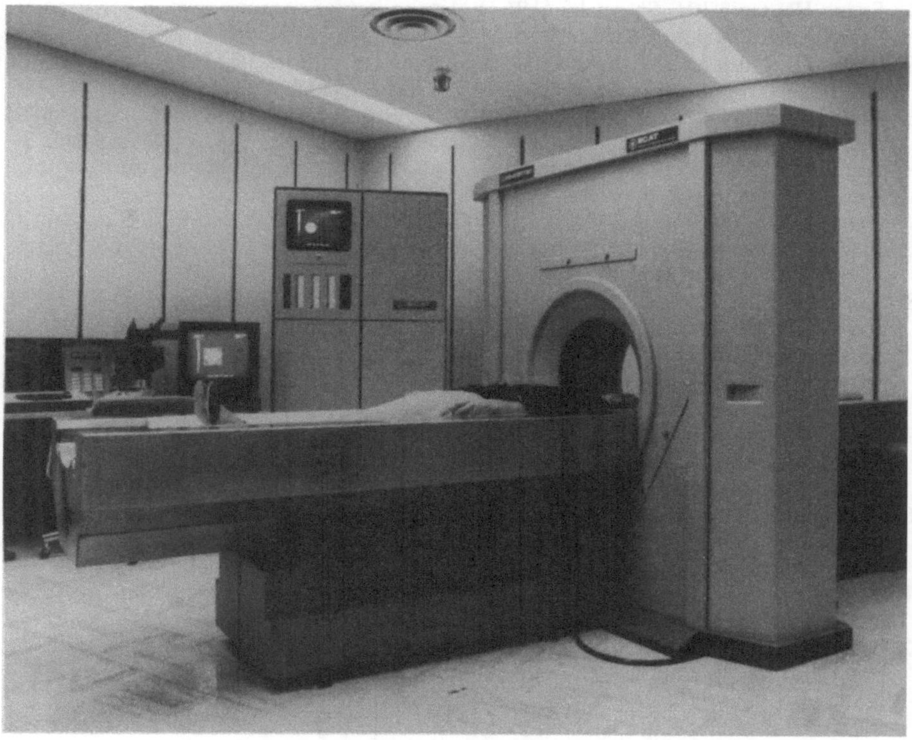

Fig. 14. Emission-computerized, axial tomographic scanner (ORTEC; EG & G)

fibrillation with no pulse deficit. The collection time for this image was 6 min. Here also, the activity distribution in myocardium is seen to be homogeneous; both ventricles are well deliniated.

The experience obtained so far with ^{11}C-methyl glucose in five normal subjects and two patients with coronary artery disease demonstrates that this radiopharmaceutical exhibits a number of important characteristics for myocardial studies. It is rapidly taken up by the myocardium and has sufficient tissue retention. These properties indicate that MG might, in future, provide a unique tool for in vivo assessment of the state and function of myocardial cell membrane. The elucidation of this possibility is the aim of our future studies.

References

1 Ballard FB, Danfarth WH, Neagle S, Bing RJ (1960) Myocardial metabolism of fatty acids. J Clin Invest 39:717–721

2 Cheung JY, Conover C, Regen DM, Whitfield CF, Morgan HE (1973) Effect of insulin on kinetics of sugar transport in heart muscle. Am J Physiol 250:E70–E78

3 Daus HJ, Reske SN, Vyska K, Feinendegen LE (1980) Pharmacokinetics of ω-[p-^{131}I-phenil]-pentadecanoic acid in heart. 18th international annual meeting of european society of nuclear medicine, Nürnberg, September 9–12

4 Evans JR, Opie LH, Shipp JC (1963) Metabolism of palmitic acid in perfused rat heart. Am J Physiol 205:766–770

5 Evans JR, Gunton RW, Baker RG, Beanlands DS, Spears JC (1965) Use of radioiodinated fatty acids for photoscans of the heart. Circ Res 16:1–10

6 Freundlieb, Höck A, Vyska K, Machula HJ, Stoecklin G, Feinendegen LE (1978) Nuklearmedizinische Analysen des Fettsäureumsatzes im Myokard. In: Oeff K, Schmidt HAE (eds) Nuklearmedizin und Biokybernetik. Medicoinformationsdienste, Berlin, pp 415–419

7 Freundlieb C, Höck A, Vyska K, Feinendegen LE, Machula HJ, Stoecklin G (1980) Myocardial imaging and metabolic studies with [17-^{123}I]-iodoheptadecanoic acid. J Nucl Med 21:1043–2050

8 Gallagher BM, Ansari A, Atkins H, Casella V, Christman DR, Fowler JS, Ido T (1977) Radiopharmaceuticals. XXVII. ^{18}F-labeled 2-deoxy-2-fluoro-D-glucose as a radiopharmaceutical for measuring regional myocardial glucose metabolism in vivo: tissue distribution and imaging studies in animals. J Nucl Med 18:990–996

9 Höck A, Freundlich C, Vyska K, Loesse B, Erbel R, Feinendegen LE (1980) The metabolism of ω-^{123}I-heptadecanoic acid in patients with heart disease (Abstract). J Nucl Med 21:90

10 Hoffman EJ, Phelps ME, Weiss ES, Welsh MJ, Coleman RE, Sobel BE, Ter-Pogossian MM (1977) Transaxial tomographic imaging of canine myocardium with ^{11}C-palmitic acid. Nucl Med 18:57–61

11 Idell-Wenger JA, Grotyohan LW, Neely JR (1978) Coenzyme A and carnitine distribution in normal and ischemic hearts. J Biol Chem 25:4310–4318

12 Ido T, Wan CN, Fowler JS, Gutterson J, Wolf AP (1977) Fluorination with F_2. A convenient synthesis of ^{18}F-2-deoxyfluoro-D-glucose. J Org Chem 42:2341–2342

13 Kloster G, Müller-Platz C, Laufer P (1980) 3-[^{11}C]-Methyl-D-glucose a potential agent for regional cerebral glucose utilisation studies (Abstract). In: Riccabona G, Schmidt HAE (eds) Clinical Significance of Nuclear Medicine. F.K. Schattauer, Stuttgart New York, pp 210–213

14 Lambrecht RM, Martinek R, Wolf AP (to be published) Cyclotron isotopes and radiopharmaceuticals. XXIII. Novel anhydrous ^{18}F-fluorinating intermediates. Int J Appl Radiat Isot

15 Machulla HJ, Stoecklin G, Kufternagel Ch, Freundlieb C, Hoeck A, Vyska K, Feinendegen LE (1978) Comparative evaluation of fatty acids labeled with C-11, Cl-34m, Br-77, and I-123 for metabolic studies of the myocardium: concise communication. J Nucl Med 19:298–302

16 Miller HI, Gold M, Spitzer JJ (1962) Removal and mobilization of individual free fatty acids in dogs. Am J Physiol 202:370–379

17 Nakahara HT, Özand P (1963) Studies of tissue permeability. IX. The effect of insulin on the penetration of 3-Methylglucose in frog muscle. J Biol Chem 238: 4P–9P
18 Phelphs ME, Hoffman EJ, Selin C, Huang SC, Robinson G, MacDonald N, Schubert H (1978) Investigation of [^{18}F] ω-2-fluoro-2-deoxyglycuse for the measure of myocardial glucose metabolism. J Nucl Med 19:1311–1319
19 Poe ND, Robinson GD, MacDonald NS (1975) Myocardial extraction of labeled long-chain fatty acid analogues. Proc Soc Exp Biol Med 148:215–218
20 Poe ND, Robinson GDJ, Graham LS, MacDonald NS (1976) Experimental basis for myocardial imaging with ^{123}I-labeled hexadecanoic acid. J Nucl Med 17: 1077–1082
21 Reeves J (1975) Stimulation of 3-0-Methylglucose transport by aerobiosos in rat thymocoytes. J Biol Chem 250:9413–9420
22 Robinson GD, Lee AW (1975) Radioiodinated fatty acids for heart imaging: Iodine monochloride addition compared with iodine replacement labeling. J Nucl Med 16:17–21
23 Rothlin ME, Bing RJ (1961) Extraction and release of individual free fatty acids by the heart and fat depots. J Clin Invest 40:1380–1386
24 Sobel BE (1979) Assuming the current needs of cardiology (Abstract). J Nucl Med 20:589
25 Stein O, Stein Y (1963) Metabolism of fatty acids in the isolated perfused heart. Biochem Biophys Acta 70:517–530
26 Stein O, Stein Y (1968) Lipid synthesis, intracellular transport and storage III. Electronmicroscopic radioautographic study of the rat heart perfused with tritiated oleic acid. J Cell Biol 36:63–77
27 Stratmann M, Welch MJ (1973) The liquid chromatographic purification of carbon -11 labeled glucose. Int Appl Radiat Isot 24:234–236
28 Vyska K, Höck A, Freundlieb C, Profant H, Feinendegen LE, Machula HJ, Stoecklin G (1979) Myocardial imaging and measurement of myocardial fatty acid metabolism using ω-I-123-heptadecanoic acid (Abstract). J Nucl Med 20:650
29 Vyska K, Höck A, Freundlieb C, Feinendegen LE, Kloster G, Stoecklin G (1980) (3-C^{11})-Methylglucose; a promising agent for in vivo assessment of function of myocardial cell membrane. J Nucl Med 21:P56–P57
30 Weiss ES, Hoffman EJ, Phelps ME, Welch MJ, Ter Pogossian MM, Sobel BE (1975) External detection of altered metabolism of ^{11}C-labeled substrates in ischemic myocardium. Clin Res 23:383A
31 Weiss ES, Hoffman EJ, Phelps ME, Welch MJ, Henry PD, Ter Pogossian MM, Sobel BE (1976) External detection and visualisation of myocardial ischemia with ^{11}C-substrates in vitro and in vivo. Circ Res 39:24–32
32 Whitesell RR, Gliemann J (1979) Kinetic parameters of transport of 3-0-Methylglucose and glucose in adipocytes. J Biol Chem 25:5276–5283

Exercise and Myocardial Ischemia in Patients with Angina Pectoris*

A.P. Selwyn, K.M. Fox, R. Allan, A. Jonathan, and T. Jones

Introduction

The majority of individuals with coronary atherosclerosis do not develop clinical coronary heart disease. The clinical manifestations of angina pectoris are highly variable and the clinician needs to know more about the relationships between myocardial ischemia, chest pain, the causes of ischemia, and the factors that cause the progression and complication of coronary atherosclerosis [2, 5, 6].

This research is concerned with using 16-point precordial mapping of the ECG during exercise and Holter monitoring of the ECG to detect the frequency of myocardial ischemia and its relation to chest pain. A short-lived isotope (krypton-81m) has been used to assess changes in regional myocardial perfusion during ischemia and to look for any systematic differences between ischemia during atrial pacing and during exercise.

Methods

Eighteen patients presented consecutively to the Hammersmith Hospital with daily angina pectoris. These patients were selected for study and underwent the following procedures:

1. Sixteen-point precordial mapping of the electrocardiogram was performed before, during, and after a maximum symptom-limited exercise test using a bicycle ergometer [3].
2. Two electrocardiographic recordings, both taken over a 24-h period, were made while the patient was ambulant. This was done using a medilog 2 FM recorder, a cassette, and a medilog 2 ST segment analyzer [7].
3. Coronary and left ventricular angiocardiography were performed using the Judkins technique.
4. Myocardial scintigraphy using a continuous infusion of krypton-81m into the right and left aortic sinuses was conducted. A gamma camera and digital computer were used to record quantitative frames every 30 s before, during, and after a standardized atrial pacing test and also straight leg raising for 5 min [8, 9].

* This research was supported in part by the British Heart Foundation and the Wellcome Trust

Results

During the exercise test the heart rate increased from 75 ± 10 beats per minute to 161 ± 19 beats per minute and the systolic blood pressure increased from 124 mm Hg (mean) to 183 mm Hg (mean). The patients achieved 34 000 ± 7 000 J. All of the patients experienced angina pectoris during the exercise test and showed a total of 12 ± 4 mm of significant ST segment depression immediately after exercise.

The Holter ECG tape recordings showed that each patient experienced 14 ± 10 episodes of significant ST segment depression during each 24-h period. Of these episodes, 16% were associated with anginal chest pain and 21% were associated with a heart rate increase of less than 10% and/or a heart rate that was ⩽ 70 beats per minute.

The coronary arteriography showed stenosis (⩾ 70%) of at least one major coronary artery in all the patients.

The krypton scintigraphy showed stable regional myocardial perfusion (less than ± 5%) before atrial pacing or exercise in all the patients. Each patient also showed a remote segment of ventricular myocardium that increased perfusion during the atrial pacing (83 ± 15.0%). All 18 patients also showed an area of ventricular myocardium that did no increase perfusion at the onset of atrial pacing and during pacing developed a progressive decrease in regional myocardial perfusion (74 ± 11%) that preceded ST segment depression, by 140 ± 80 s. This absolute decrease of regional myocardial

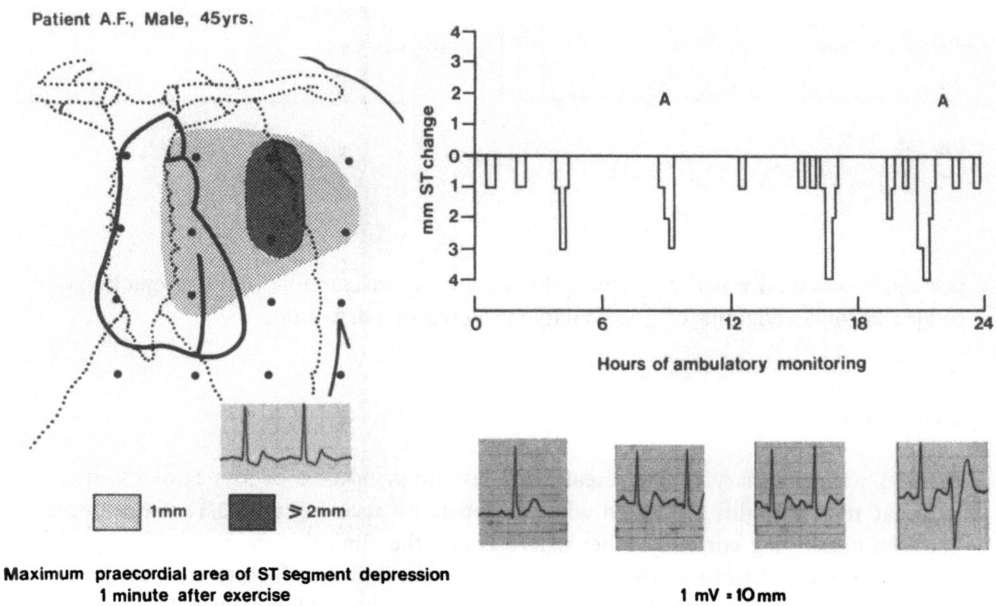

Fig. 1a, b. Results of a 24-h electrocardiographic recording in an ambulatory patient with angina pectoris. The tracings show that ST segment depression occurs more frequently than angina pectoris. Significant ST depression also occurs at night and with no increase in heart rate. These findings raise questions about the cause of myocardial ischemia

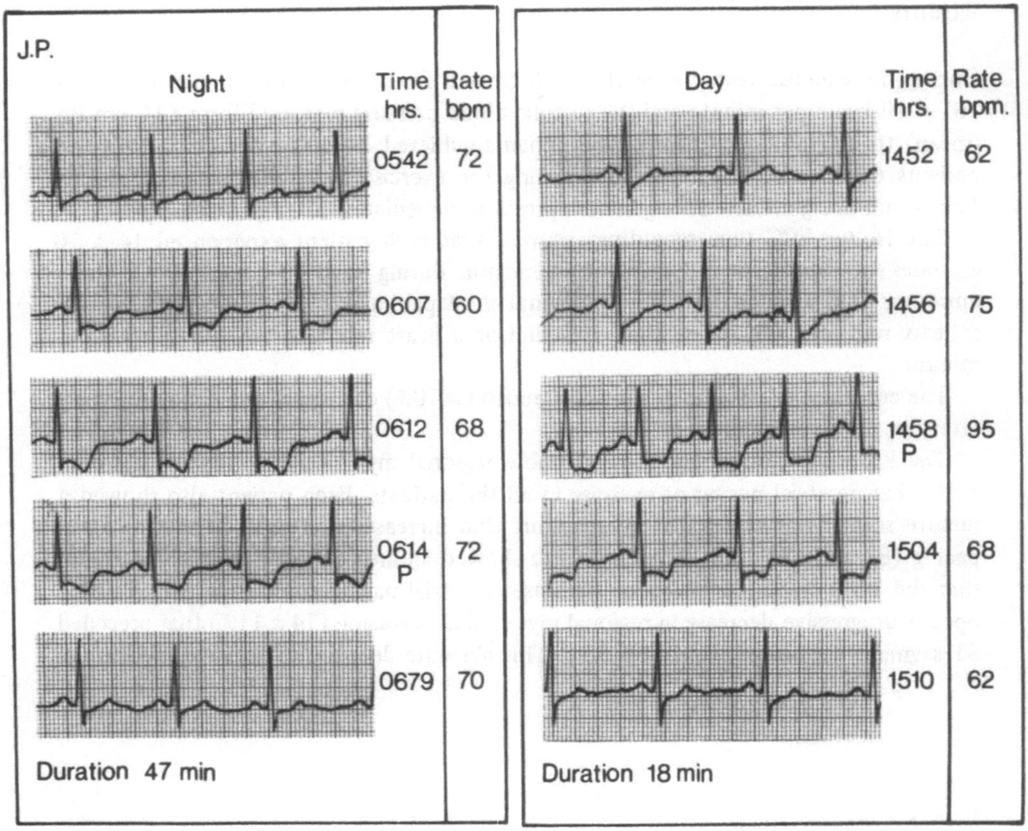

Fig. 1b

perfusion was confirmed in seven patients by reconstruction of 64 projections in single photon tomograms using calculated attenuation correction.

Discussion

Patients with coronary artery disease can develop symptoms of myocardial ischemia while at rest, at night, and often with no apparent preceding cause. The relationship between underlying coronary atherosclerosis and the clinical state is complicated and not direct and, therefore, the causes of ischemia and the factors that complicate coronary artery disease are of clinical and pathophysiological importance [1, 4, 5, 7].

This work shows that patients suffer many asymptomatic episodes of myocardial ischemia. The relationship between chest pain and ischemia is inconsistent and a proportion of events occur with no increase in heart rate. This raises important questions: What mechanisms trigger the ischemic events? Is the objective evidence of myocardial ischemia the best measure of efficacy when assessing the effect of treatments?

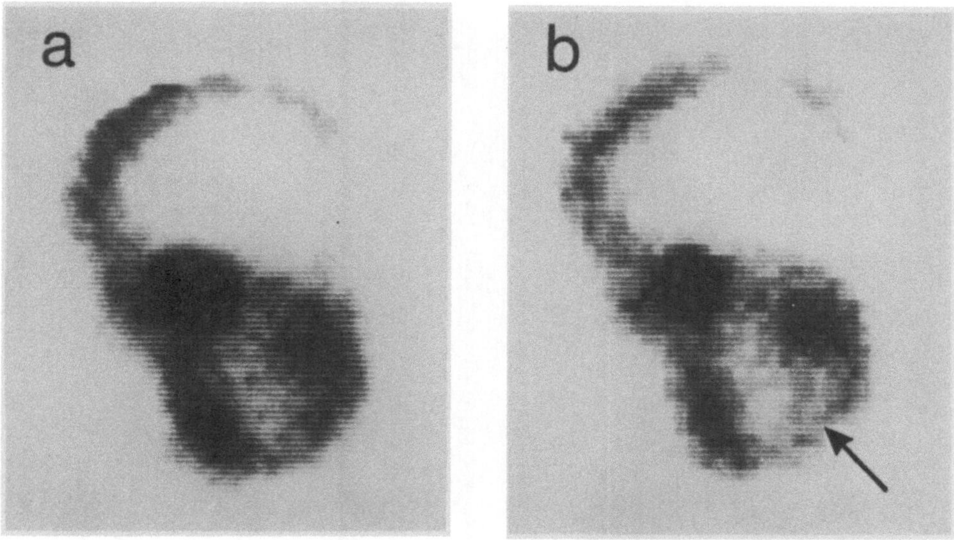

Fig. 2. These scintigrams were recorded from a patient with angina pectoris and significant stenosis of three major coronary arteries. The first scintigram recorded at rest shows delivery of the tracer to the aortic sinuses and the distribution of regional myocardial perfusion (**a**). During pacing there is an absolute decrease of regional myocardial perfusion preceding ST segment depression and chest pain (**b**)

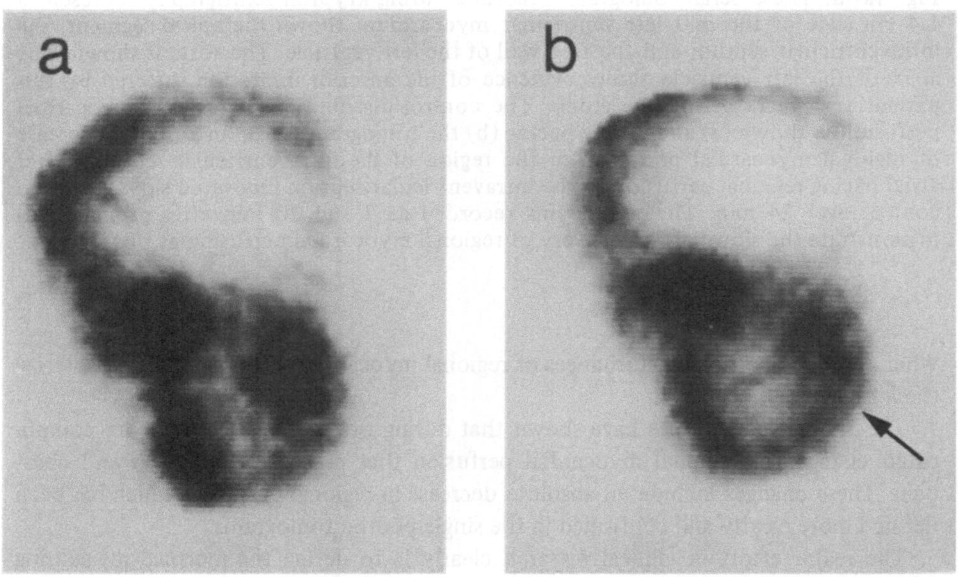

Fig. 3. These scintigrams were recorded from the same patient shown in Fig. 2. The distribution of regional myocardial perfusion is shown at rest (**a**), and during leg exercises (**b**). The same absolute decrease of regional myocardial perfusion and sequence of events were recorded. The resolution was relatively poor due to patient movement

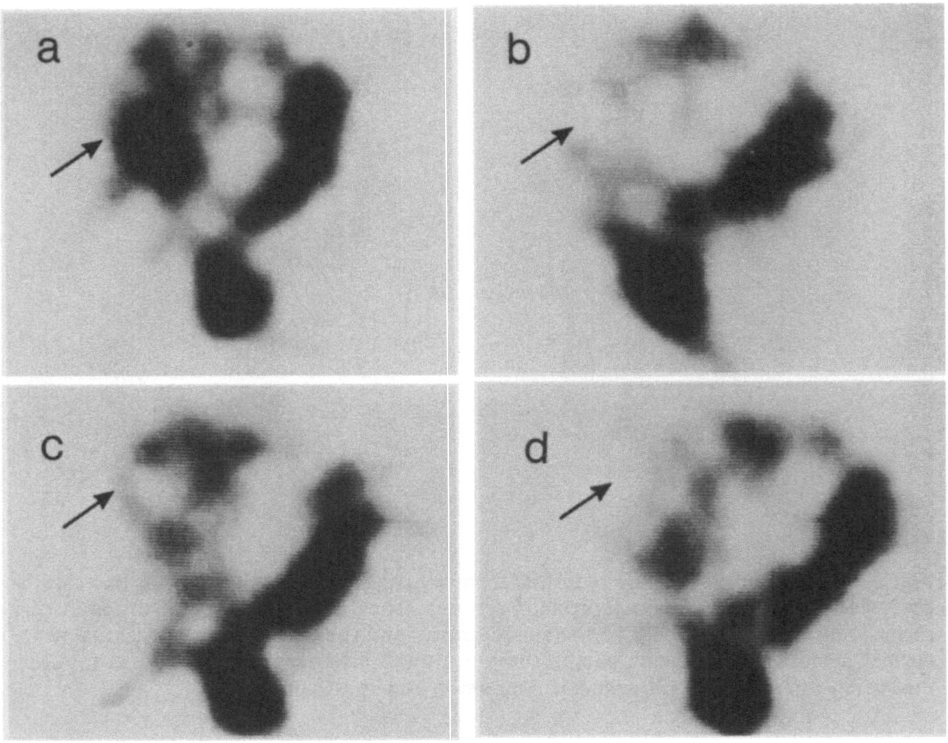

Fig. 4a–d. These serial tomograms recorded during krypton scintigraphy represent a 1.4 cm slice of the mid left ventricular myocardium shown the apical segment, the intraventricular septum and the free wall of the left ventricle. The aorta is shown. The apex of the left ventricle shows evidence of old anterior infarction suffered by this patient two years before the study. The control distribution of regional myocardial perfusion is shown (**a**) and during pacing (**b**) the tomograms show an absolute decrease of regional myocardial perfusion in the region of the intraventricular septum. After atrial pacing regional perfusion to the intraventricular septum recovered slowly back to control over 24 min. The scintigrams recorded at 7 and 20 min after pacing (**c**, **d**) demonstrate the slow partial recovery of regional myocardial perfusion at this time

What are the underlying disturbances of regional myocardial perfusion that characterize these ischemic attacks?

The short-lived isotopes have shown that during ischemic events there are complicated changes in regional myocardial perfusion that precede ST changes and chest pain. These changes include an absolute decrease in regional perfusion which has been defined more clearly and confirmed in the single-photon tomograms.

The major effort in clinical research clearly is to define the mechanisms causing these ischemic events and the relative importance of atherosclerosis and functional factors in causing myocardial ischemia and angina pectoris. The objective methods outlined with rational treatment based on these mechanisms may be used to prevent ischemia and possibly the progression of atherosclerosis.

Summary

Patients presenting with angina pectoris have undergone 16-point precordial mapping of the electrocardiogram, 24-h Holter recording of the electrocardiogram, and a study of regional myocardial perfusion (RMP) using krypton-81m and a gamma camera. This was carried out to detect myocardial ischemia and to examine the frequency and distribution of ischemic events within the myocardium.

The precordial mapping on exercise demonstrated the projection of ECG signs of ischemia and the position of maximum ST depression. This position on the chest was used for the Holter monitoring over 24 h which showed that angina pectoris accompanied only 16% of ischemic episodes and ischemic events occurred while the patients were at rest or asleep. The isotope perfusion studies during pacing and leg exercise showed absolute regional decrease of myocardial perfusion that preceded episodes of ischemic ECG signs and angina chest pain.

References

1 Baroldi A (1978) Coronary stenosis; ischaemic or non-ischaemic factors? Am Heart J 96:139
2 Enos WF, Holmes RF, Beyer JC (1953) Coronary disease among United States soldiers in action in Korea. JAMA 152:1090
3 Fox KM, Selwyn AP, Shillingford JP (1979) Precordial electrocardiographic mapping after exercise in the diagnosis of coronary artery disease. Am J Cardiol 43:541
4 Goldstein RE, Epstein SE (1972) Medical management of patients with angina pectoris. Prog Cardiovasc Dis 14:360
5 Maseri A (1972) Pathophysiological, diagnostic and methodological problems in the study of myocardial blood flow in ischaemic heart disease. J Nucl Biol Med 16:259
6 Ross RS (1975) Ischaemic heart disease, an overview. Am J of Cardiol 36:496
7 Selwyn AP, Fox KM, Ives M, Shillingford JP, Dargie H, Oaklea D (1978) Myocardial ischaemia in patients with frequent angina pectoris. Br Med J 2:1594
8 Selwyn AP, Jones T, Turner JH, Pratt T, Clark J, Lavender P (1978) Continuous assessment of regional myocardial perfusion in dogs using krypton-81m. Circ Res 42:771
9 Selwyn AP, Steiner R, Kivisaaria A, Fox KM, Forse G (1979) Krypton-81m in the physiological assessment of coronary artery stenosis in man. Am J Cardiol 43:547

Detection of Ischemic Myocardium with Exercise: Coronary Blood Flow Measurements*

W. Kübler, D. Opherk, and H. Zebe

Introduction

The evaluation of the severity of coronary heart disease and its consequences on coronary flow by eyeball assessment of coronary anatomy visualized by coronary arteriography is not a precise method: The judgment of the degree of a stenosis is subjective and its hemodynamic consequences can only roughly be estimated because of the nonlinear and nonidentical complex relationship between narrowing of the lumen and flow.

The determination of coronary blood flow in a given myocardial area would, therefore, be of the greatest importance – especially under conditions of increased flow, e.g. during exercise.

At the beginning of the last decade, Holmberg et al. [4] and Lichtlen et al. [6] reported exercise-induced changes in global coronary flow in patients with coronary heart disease; in 1977 Lichtlen [5] presented a study on regional myocardial blood flow during exercise showing a reduction in flow in the poststenotic area.

Despite these studies and despite the theoretical interest and the great clinical implications, the determination of coronary flow is far from being a routine method in the evaluation of coronary heart disease. This is due to as yet unsolved technical, methodological, and biological problems. These problems have, therefore, to be first discussed briefly, as they may account for errors up to 100% and more – especially under the conditions of exercise-induced increased flow.

Technical Problems

For quantitative determination of coronary flow either the coronary arteries or the coronary sinus has to be intubated; this is more difficult during dynamic exercise.

Methodological Problems

All indirect methods for the determination of coronary blood flow used in man are based on Ficks principle:

* Supported by a grant from the Deutsche Forschungsgemeinschaft – SFB 90 "Kardiovaskuläres System", University of Heidelberg

$$F/W = 100\,\lambda \frac{\Delta Cv}{\int_0^t (Ca\text{-}Cv)dt}$$

F/W, flow/weight [ml/100 g · min]; λ, partition coefficient; *t*, time [min]; and *Ca* and *Cv*, arterial and venous tracer concentration.

An exercise-induced increase in coronary flow leads to a decrease in the denominator, i.e., the mean arterio-coronary venous difference in tracer concentration. Hence, any error in sampling and quantification of the tracer is augmented under the conditions of exercise.

In the nominator the total in-venous tracer concentration is given as a measure of the change in myocardial tracer concentration. It is a crucial requirement for valid application of Fick's principle that the tracer concentration in the tissue, i.e., the nominator of the equation, is identical throughout the area under study. This, however, is not the case in patients with coronary heart disease, as may be seen from the results in Fig. 1. On the ordinate the arteriocoronary venous difference in percentage of the arterial concentration after 5 min of application of the easily diffusible inert gas argon is given, while on the abscissa coronary reserve is shown. It can be seen, that in patients with coronary heart disease (group I) due to heterogeneity of flow, arteriocoronary venous difference is increased, being further augmented by the presence of scar tissue due to myocardial infarction (group II). Heterogeneity of flow is further precipitated by stress-induced angina and may lead to a severe overestimation of flow, mainly in techniques with bolus injection and precordial counting.

The transient ischemic areas of the myocardium, as they may exist in typical stress-induced angina, local myocardial lipid content may be augmented due to increased lipid synthesis [3]. Using an inert gas with high fat solubility (such as, e.g., Xenon) leads to a severe underestimation of flow, because under these conditions the partition coefficient λ is erroneously assumed too low.

A further crucial requirement for the use of tracers to measure myocardial blood flow is free, not rate-limiting, diffusion into the myocardium. As the diffusion constant D is inversely related to the square root of the molecular weight M

$$D = \frac{c}{\sqrt{M}} \qquad (c\text{, constant}),$$

tracers with a higher molecular weight may lead to an underestimation of flow because of limited diffusion, especially under the conditions of exercise.

This mechanism is, e.g., discussed for Xenon.

Biological Problems

Coronary artery disease is a patchy disease. Therefore, measurements of global coronary flow, e.g., with the argon method, are only of rather limited value. In this aspect, techniques which allow the determination of regional flow, such as the Xenon residue technique, are definitely better. But is has to be kept in mind that even this technique gives only a two-dimensional picture of a three-dimensional structure. Hence, the flow in the endocardial layers, which are predominantly affected by stress-induced angina cannot be quantitated by any method nowadays in use; in the future this might be possible by use of positron-emitting computer tomography.

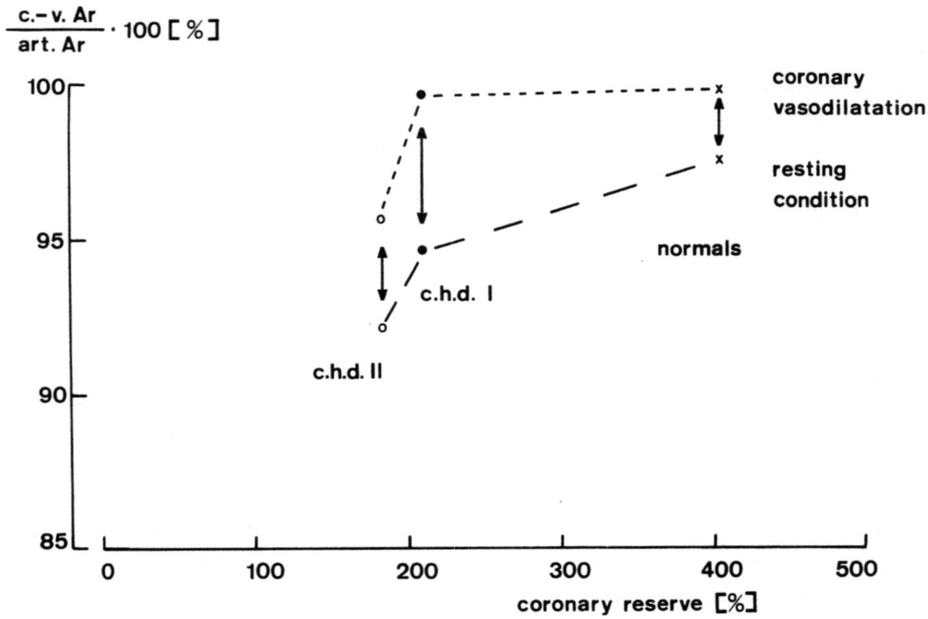

Fig. 1. The arteriocoronary venous difference in (%) of the arterial concentration (*ordinate*) after 5 min of inhalation of the easily diffusible inert gas argon for three groups of patients with differences in coronary reserve (*abscissa*).
Group 1; normals; group 2; patients with coronary heart disease (CHD I), i.e., stenosis of ⩾ 75% but no previous myocardial infarction; group 3; patients with coronary heart disease (CHD II), i.e., stenosis of ⩾ 75% and previous transmural myocardial infarction. – – – – – –, resting conditions; ––––––, after maximal coronary vasodilatation due to dipyridamole (0.5 mg/kg)

According to data obtained in animals by Bretschneider [2] and Lochner [7] and in man by Tauchert [8] maximal myocardial oxygen consumption amounts to about 30 ml/100 g per min. Under physiological conditions this value is far exceeded by maximal myocardial oxygen delivery which amounts to approximately 60 ml O_2/100 g per min. It is due to this reserve capacity in myocardial oxygen delivery that people such as Reinhold Messner and Peter Habeler can climb even Mount Everest without artificial oxygen breathing and with an arterial pO_2 of less than 50 mm Hg but no anginal pain.

As maximal myocardial oxygen delivery exceeds maximal myocardial oxygen consumption, a reduction in myocardial flow reserve does not necessarily imply myocardial ischemia, i.e., insufficient oxygen delivery compared with oxygen demands, which may in addition be reduced locally due to the presence of scar tissue.

Our own studies were performed using the argon method which, however, allows only the determination of global flow. In Fig. 2 values of myocardial blood flow under different conditions are given for normal persons and for patients with coronary heart disease. The data reveal yet another biologic and ethical problem: it is not possible to keep a patient in a state of myocardial ischemia and hence with anginal pain for some period of time just in order to obtain correct sampling of the tracer from the coronary

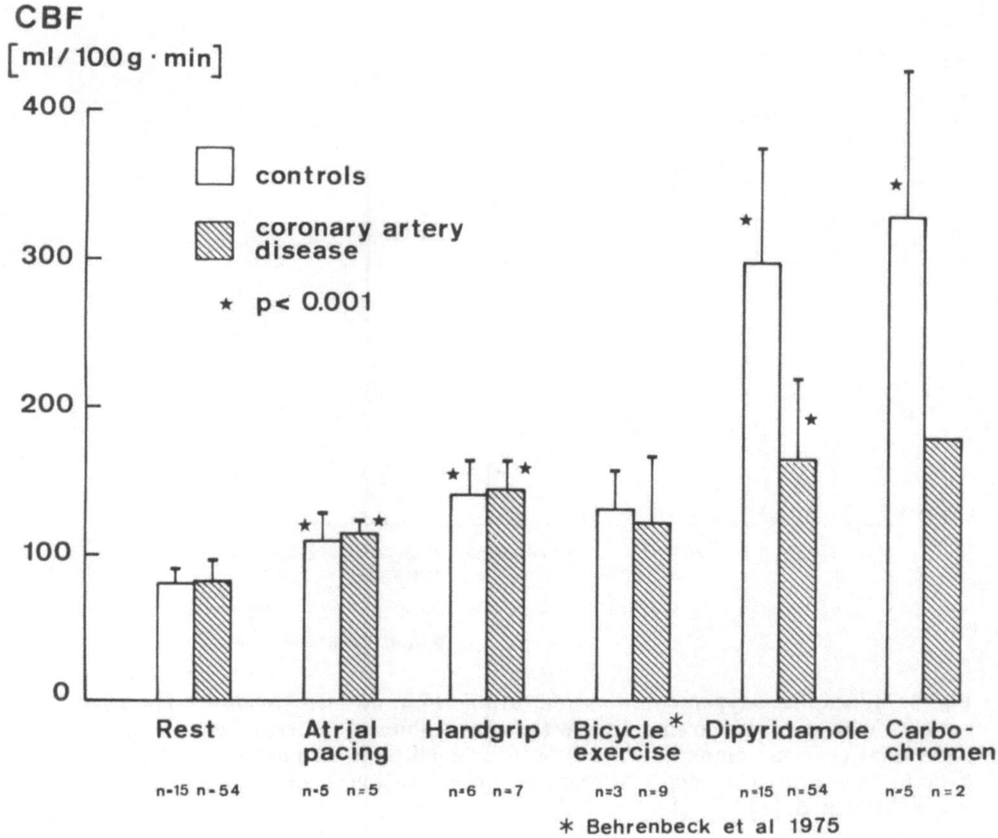

Fig. 2. Global myocardial blood flow (*ordinate*) in normals (*open columns*) and in patients with coronary artery disease (*hatched columns*) under different conditions. Only after application of coronary dilating drugs (dipyridamole) could a significant ($P < 0.001$) difference be found between the controls and the patients group. Significant changes compared with the resting conditions are characterized by *. The data for coronary flow during bicycle ergometry are taken from Behrenbeck et al. [1]

sinus. Therefore, no significant difference could be found between normals and the patients group, either during arterial pacing or during handgrip or – according to data of Behrenbeck et al. [1] – during bicycle ergometry.

However, by application of selective coronary dilating drugs (such as dipyridamole or carbochromen), a marked difference can be found with relative reduction of flow in the patient group. This approach, therefore, seems to be the best and the safest for the determination of coronary reserve.

The reduction in flow response is independent of myocardial oxygen demands, which are highest under dynamic and isometric (handgrip) exercise and lowest after carbochromen despite an increase in flow by about 400% (Fig. 3).

Figure 4 reveals the relationship between coronary reserve, given on the ordinate, and the severity of the sclerotic lesions – seen on the coronary angiogram and quantitated by the Gensini score – given on the abscissa. A rather logarithmic relationship

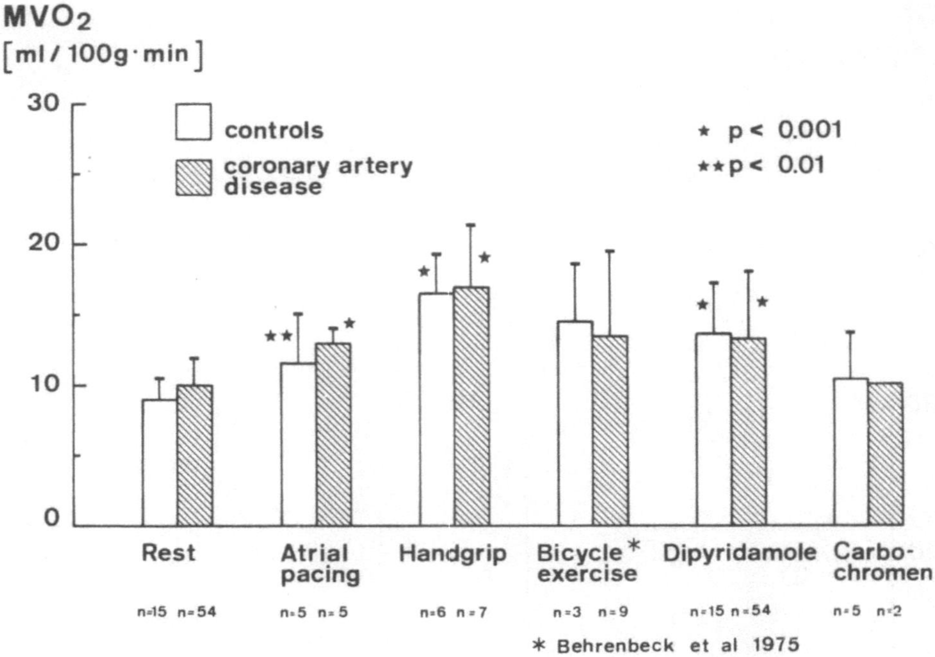

Fig. 3. Myocardial oxygen consumption (*ordinate*) in normals (*open columns*) and in patients with coronary artery disease (*hatched columns*) under different conditions. Significant changes compared with the resting conditions are characterized by *. The data for myocardial oxygen consumption during bicycle ergometry are taken from Behrenbeck et al. [1]

is obtained, this being due to methodological problems related to nonhomogeneous flow and to the presence of scar tissue with reduced oxygen demands.

The relationship between coronary reserve on the ordinate and left ventricular function – given as the ejection fraction on the abscissa – is shown in Fig. 5. Based on the determination of coronary reserve, there is clear separation between normals (open circles) and the patient groups. As can be anticipated from data presented earlier, there is a nonlinear, rather parabolic function between coronary reserve and left ventricular function.

Although the determination of global coronary reserve, or (as shown by Lichtlen [5]) of regional flow during dynamic exercise allows a rather clear separation between normals and patients with coronary heart disease, both methods are far from being used under routine conditions and generally not very helpful as diagnostic procedures.

There might, however, be one exception, in which the determination of the coronary dilatory capacity might be of diagnostic help, i.e., syndrome X. This comprises patients with a history of typical stress-induced angina promptly relieved by nitroglycerin, a pathologic resting and/or exercise ECG but a normal coronary angiogram, normal left ventricular function at rest but impairment during exercise and, as seen on biopsy specimens, degenerative changes of myocardial cells but unchanged intramyocardial small vessels. In these patients a significant and pronounced reduction in

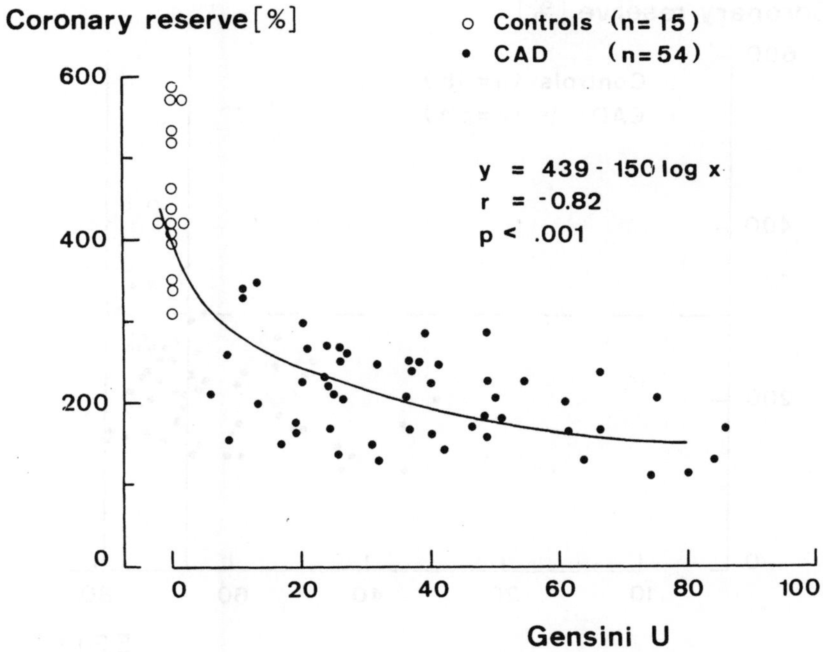

Fig. 4. The relationship between the severity of the sclerotic lesions seen on the coronary angiogram and quantitated by the Gensini score (*abscissa*) and coronary reserve (*ordinate*). Normals, *open circles*. Patients with coronary artery disease, *heavy dots*. $y = 439-150 \log x; r = 0.82; P < 0.001$

coronary reserve – like in patients with severe sclerotic lesions – can be observed (Table 1).

Conclusions

1. The determination of myocardial blood flow – especially in patients with coronary heart disease and nonhomogeneity of the myocardium and its perfusion – has still several unsolved methodological problems.
2. As coronary reserve and hence maximal myocardial oxygen delivery greatly exceeds maximal myocardial oxygen consumption, a reduction or inadequate response in coronary flow, especially to conditions of increased flow, does not necessarily indicate myocardial ischemia.
3. In patients with coronary heart disease under conditions of increased flow a reduction in the flow response can be observed; the greater the increase in flow rate, the greater the difference between normals and the patients group.
4. At present, measurements of coronary blood flow may be helpful in the clinical diagnosis of patients with syndrome X, i.e., patients with typical angina but a normal coronary angiogram. The disorder is characterized by a greatly reduced coronary reserve of about 50%.

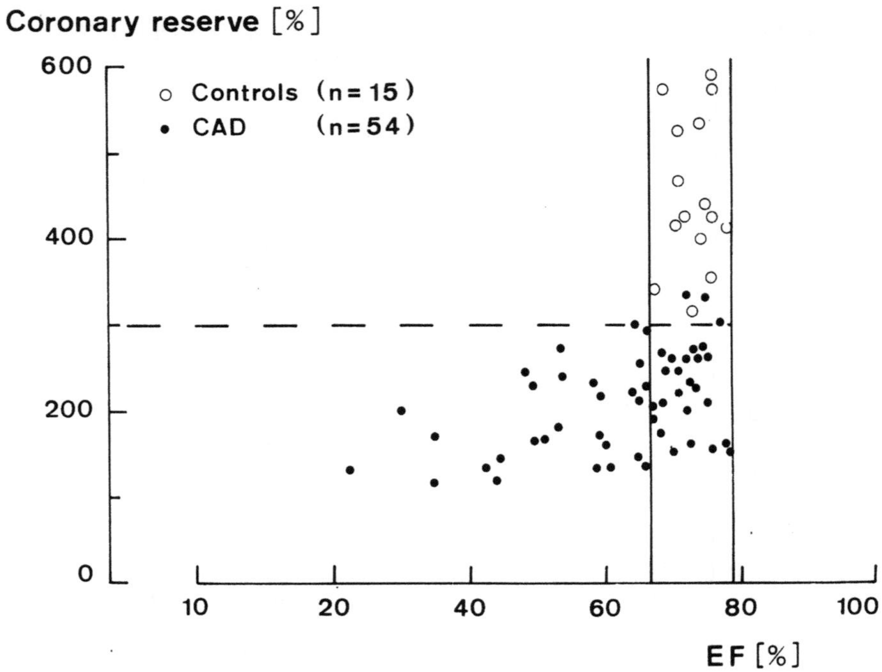

Fig. 5. The relationship between the ejection fraction (*EF*) given on the *abscissa* and coronary reserve (*ordinate*) for controls (*open circles*) and patients with coronary artery disease with and without previous myocardial infarction (*heavy dots*). The *horizontal broken line* indicates the border between normals and patients with coronary artery disease. The determination of coronary reserve enables a rather clear separation of normals from the patient group. The *hatched column* signifies the normal range of the *EF*; it does not allow a separation between controls and CAD

Table 1. Sclerotic lesions seen on the angiogram and quantitated by the Gensini score, left ventricular (LV) function given as the ejection fraction (EF), and coronary reserve for five different groups of patients

		n	Gensini score (u)	LV function EF (%)	Coronary reserve (%)
Controls[a]		15	0	73 ± 3.1	452 ± 89.1
CHD	Group I[b]	24	26 ± 15.1	72 ± 3.8	237 ± 61.3*
	Group II[c]	30	47 ± 19.7	55 ± 12.5*	190 ± 46.7*
Angina pectoris but normal coronary arteries (syndrome X)[d]		21	0	72 ± 4.5	224 ± 49.5*

* $P < 0.001$

[a] Controls: no sclerotic lesions (Gensini score: 0), normal LV function and normal coronary reserve.

Table 1 (continued)

[b] Group I: sclerotic lesions but no previous myocardial infarction and hence normal LV function, but reduced coronary reserve.

[c] Group II: sclerotic lesions, previous myocardial infarction and hence reduced EF and reduced coronary reserve.

[d] No sclerotic lesions, normal EF under resting conditions, but greatly reduced coronary reserve

References

1 Behrenbeck DW, Tauchert M, Freyland MD, Niehues B, Röhrig FJ, Hilger HH (1975) Vergleich zwischen ergometrischer Belastbarkeit und medikamentös erschließbarer Koronarreserve bei Patienten mit koronarer Herzkrankheit (KHK) Verh Dtsch Ges Inn Med 65:253
2 Bretschneider HJ (1961) Sauerstoffbedarf und -versorgung des Herzmuskels. Ver Dtsch Ges Kreislaufforsch 27:32
3 Harris P (1974) Hypoxia and fat metabolism. In: Muir J (ed) Prospects in the management of ischemic heart disease. Ciba Laboratories, Horsham, p 158
4 Holmberg S, Serzysko W, Varnaushkas E (1971) Coronary circulation during heavy exercise in control subjects and patients with coronary heart disease. Acta Med Scand 190:645
5 Lichtlen P (1977) Myocardial blood flow during exercise in patients with coronary artery disease. Herz 2:31
6 Lichtlen P, Gattiker K, Scholer Y, Schibli R (1973) Koronarfluß unter Arbeit bei Koronarsklerose, gemessen anhand der präkordialen Xenon-Clearance-Technik. Ver Dtsch Ges Kreislaufforsch 39:301
7 Lochner W (1965) Substratumsatz, Sauerstoffverbrauch und anaerober Energiegewinn des Herzens. Z Kreislaufforsch 54:103
8 Tauchert M (1973) Koronarreserve und maximaler Sauerstoffverbrauch des menschlichen Herzens. Basic Res Cardiol 68:183

MIX
Papier aus verantwortungsvollen Quellen
Paper from responsible sources
FSC® C105338

If you have any concerns about our products,
you can contact us on
ProductSafety@springernature.com

In case Publisher is established outside the EU,
the EU authorized representative is:
Springer Nature Customer Service Center GmbH
Europaplatz 3, 69115 Heidelberg, Germany

Printed by Libri Plureos GmbH
in Hamburg, Germany